A HEALTHY FUTURE

Educating children in preventative healthcare

I0122732

by

Rabbi Avraham Greenbaum

Edited by Nachum Shaw

Promised Land

JERUSALEM   LONDON   NEW YORK

For further information:

Promised Land Publishers

Apt. 8, 5 Gimmel Alroyi St.

Jerusalem 9210808

ISRAEL

or

Promised Land Publishers

8 Woodville Road

London NW11 9TN

ENGLAND

or

Promised Land Publishers

67 Wood Hollow Lane

New Rochelle

NY 10804

USA

Email: promisedland920@gmail.com

www.promisedlandpublishers.com

CONTENTS

A HEALTHY FUTURE

Educating children in preventative healthcare

by

Rabbi Avraham Greenbaum

"And He said, 'If you will listen carefully to the voice of God and do what is right in His eyes and give ear to His precepts and keep all His statutes, I will put none of the diseases upon you that I have put on the Egyptians. For I, God am your Healer' "

EXODUS 15:26

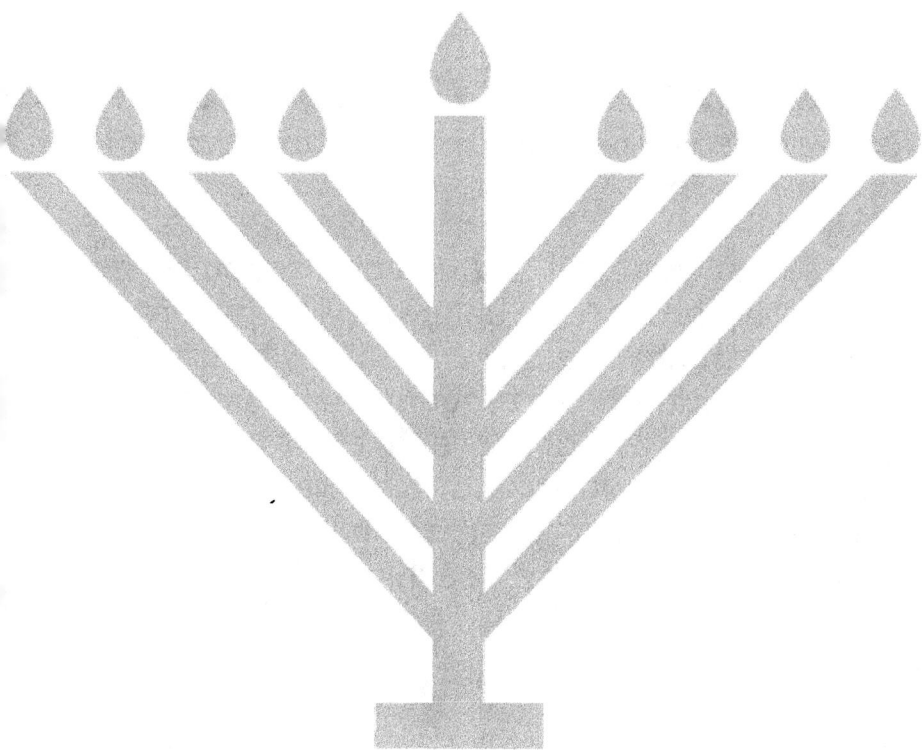

A Healthy Future

Educating children in preventative healthcare

"Done beautifully in good taste and with wisdom." -- HaRav Ovadia Yosef z"l

"This book deserves a place in every Jewish home and every Torah educational institution." -- Dr. Geoffrey Greenfield, Pediatrician, Jerusalem

1 Contemporary Health Hazards
Why preventive healthcare is more vital today than ever before

We live in a world of technological sophistication and material prosperity unknown in any previous era. The benefits are very many, yet prosperity and sophistication have brought many problems of their own. Our way of life and environment pose serious threats to our health and wellbeing. Today it's more vital than ever to help our children protect their health by teaching them to make healthy choices as they find their way in this confusing world.

Food & Diet

Revolutionary methods of agriculture, food production, preservation, refrigeration, transport and marketing have made an abundance of food products of every kind readily available to large sections of the population. Supermarket shelves are stacked with a bewildering array of choices.

Many people's diet includes a high proportion of snacks and fast foods.

Too much fat and sugar

The average diet in many "advanced" countries is too high in fats and sugars, causing obesity and increasing the risk of heart disease, the leading killer in the "advanced" countries.

Malnutrition without hunger?

Many people rely on foods that do not provide them with the right balance of vital nutrients. A diet rich in the wrong ingredients can be a poor diet for the body and may cause impaired physical and mental functioning and increase the risk of serious illnesses, including osteoporosis, diabetes and cancer.

What's in it and what will it do to me?
Contemporary agriculture relies heavily on fertilizers, growth aids, pesticides and genetic engineering. Food manufacture often involves removal of many natural food components while artificial preservatives, flavorings, coloring, vitamins, minerals and other substances are added. In many cases, the effects on health of contemporary processes and additives are unknown.

Mental, emotional and behavioral problems
Experts point to poor nutrition as a significant factor in many mental, emotional and behavioral

problems among youth today, including hyperactivity, attention deficit, mood swing, aggression and violence.

In a world of multiple food options, it's vital to teach our children to make good choices.

Technology

At home and at work, technology has made our lives physically much easier. Cars and elevators save us the need to walk and climb stairs. Tasks that used to involve considerable physical effort are today performed at the push of a button by phones, computers and countless other inventions.

Recipe for obesity

When people are physically inactive but eat too rich a diet, they get fat! Inadequate physical activity can lead to loss of muscle strength, joint flexibility and bone strength as well as many other problems.

When normal everyday activities are physically undemanding, some form of exercise is necessary to maintain health and fitness.

Hazards all around us

With all its benefits, technology has also brought many potential hazards into our lives at home and outside, from electrical outlets and appliances, flammable materials, dangerous chemicals and poisonous medicines to dangers on the roads and many more.

Teaching our children proper caution in the home and outside is a matter of survival!

Stress

Technology is supposed to save us time and effort yet it often seems to make our lives more complicated. Today's high-speed, high-pressure lifestyle with its barrage of noise, beeps, rings, flashing lights, blinking screens, vibrations, electromagnetic fields and much more puts people under tremendous stress. Stress may cause anxiety, fatigue and depression as well as many other mental, emotional, nervous and physical problems.

Good health helps protect against the adverse effects of stress. To help our children stand up to the challenges of a high-pressure world, we must teach them healthy habits.

Quality of the environment

Our sophisticated, extravagant, industry and technology-based society takes a heavy toll on the environment in which we live. Throughout the world countless tons of industrial waste, chemicals, heavy metals, radioactive substances, garbage, unsanitary waste and much more are daily dumped on land or poured into rivers and seas, causing untold damage to natural systems and resources, affecting the foods we eat and water we drink. Heavy emissions of poisonous and other gases by automobiles, industry and even home spray-cans not only pollute the air we breathe but are causing serious long-term damage to the earth's atmosphere, which is even upsetting weather patterns.

Known and unknown effects of pollution
Research indicates that various kinds of environmental pollution are directly associated with higher incidence of certain serious illnesses and other health problems in the population as a whole and especially in those sectors that are more exposed. Many other phenomena -- from allergies of various kinds to fatigue, loss of mental acuity and nervous problems -- are also thought by many to be bound up with environmental pollution.

What can we do about it?

In most cases we can't help being exposed to pollution. The surest way to protect ourselves is by leading the healthiest possible lifestyle. When people eat a poor diet, fail to take proper exercise and abuse their health in other ways, they make it harder for their bodies to cope with the assault from the outside environment.

Teaching our children healthy habits is the best way to ensure a healthy future for them and for the generations to come.

2 Guard Yourself!
The mitzvah of caring for body and soul

Our sages teach us that the true purpose for which we enter this world is to come closer to God through study of the Torah and fulfillment of its commandments. Through this our souls are elevated, attaining good in this world and forever.

The soul can only enter the physical world in the garb of the physical body. The body is the soul's instrument to attain its purpose in this world. Only through the body can we carry out the practical *mitzvos* of the Torah, which relate to things of this world.

In order to survive in the physical world we are obliged to provide the body with what it needs, such as food and drink. Enjoyment of the material world has a legitimate place in our service of God when it assists us in linking the physical with the spiritual. But when satisfaction of our material inclinations goes beyond the proper bounds, this can cause damage to the soul and the body. The soul's mission is to take control of these inclinations, directing the body to its true purpose.

To ensure that the body will be a fitting instrument with which to perform the *mitzvos*, God has commanded us to protect and guard our bodies: "Guard yourself and guard your soul very carefully" (Deuteronomy 4:9-10).

This commandment is so important that our rabbis taught that it is part of the commandment not to forget the Giving of the Torah: "Guard yourself and guard your soul very much *lest you forget. the day when you stood before HaShem Your God at Horev*" (Deuteronomy 4:9-10). The classic commentator *Kli Yakar* explains: "'Guard yourself' means taking care of the body."

Bodily health is the foundation for keeping all the commandments of the Torah since in most cases they are bound up with physical action of some kind. When the body is unfit and unhealthy, this detracts from proper fulfillment of the commandments.

In the words of *Rambam* (Maimonides): "Bodily health and wellbeing are part of the path to God, for it is impossible to understand or have any knowledge of the Creator when one is sick. Therefore, one must avoid anything that may harm the body and one must cultivate healthful habits" (*Hilchos De'os* 4:1).

> Man's use of the world for his own needs should be circumscribed by the limits imposed by God's Will and should not include anything forbidden by God. It should be motivated by the need to best maintain his health and preserve his life, and not merely to satisfy his physical urges and superfluous desires. One's motivation in maintaining his body should furthermore be so that the soul should be able to use it to serve its Creator, without being hampered by the body's weakness and incapability. When man makes use of the world in this manner, this itself becomes an act of perfection, and

through it one can attain the same virtue as in keeping the other commandments. Indeed, one of the commandments requires that we keep our bodies fit so that we can serve God, and that we derive our needs from the environment to achieve this goal. In this manner, we elevate ourselves even through such activities. The world itself is also elevated, since it is then also helping man to serve God.

-- Rabbi Moshe Chaim Luzzatto, Derech Hashem 1:4:7.

Our health is in our hands

"Everything is in the hands of heaven except chills and fevers (which sometimes come though negligence)". (*Babylonian Talmud, Kesuvos* 30a and *Rashi*.)

The time, place and circumstances in which each soul is born into this world are decreed by God. Each person has his or her own unique body and constitution. Not everyone is born with the gift of a healthy body. When we *are* born with this precious gift, we must be grateful to God for His kindness and do everything in our power to cherish and protect it.

Our health and the length and quality of our lives are to a large extent in our own hands. The body grows older every day and must eventually die. Yet proper attention to its needs and avoidance of harmful habits can increase the length and quality of our lives, saving us from many illnesses, accidents and other troubles that can strike through neglect and abuse.

"The wise person has his eyes in his head" (Koheles 2:14) -- "He sees what is ahead" (*Avos* 2:9). Good health is a precious gift, and the wise person does everything necessary to protect it from possible hazards by taking proper care of the body.

On the other hand, "The fool loses everything he is given" (*Chagiga* 4a). Our sages teach us that when a doctor heals the sick, the doctor is performing the mitzvah of returning lost property: "And you shall return it to him" (Deuteronomy 22:2) - "This refers to the loss of the person's body, i.e. his health" (*Sanhedrin* 73a; see Rambam's Commentary on *Mishnah Nedarim* 4:4).

It is better to guard your health than to have to try to get it back if God forbid you lose it.

How do we guard our health?

In much of the wider world, health is valued not only as a condition of productivity but also as one of the main keys to the enhancement and prolongation of life. Not only are enormous effort and resources poured into the promotion of health by governments, the public health and medical establishments, in education and the media. There is also a vast, lucrative health economy that spans everything from breakfast cereals and sports shoes to exotic herbal remedies and computerized fitness equipment. In practice, many people's pursuit of health goes no further than swallowing a few vitamins pills or being passive sports spectators.

The Jewish goal in the pursuit of health and our path towards it are qualitatively different. For the Jew, health is valued primarily as the essential condition for serving God through following the commandments.

Keeping the commandments is itself a guarantee against illness, as promised to the Jewish People directly after leaving Egypt and crossing the Red Sea. This was at Marah, their first camp in the wilderness, even before the Giving of the Torah at Sinai: "There He laid down for him a statute and a judgment. And He said, If you will surely listen to the voice of HaShem your God and do what is right in His eyes and attend to His commandments and guard all His statutes, *all the diseases that I have put upon the Egyptians, I will not put upon you, for I HaShem am your Healer*" (Exodus 15:26).

Serving God draws His blessing into our very food and drink, protecting our health: "And you shall serve Hashem your God, and He will bless your bread and your water, and I will remove illness from within you" (Exodus 23:25).

We keep the Torah not only because it is the means to protect our health but more essentially because this is what God has commanded us. Yet the true Torah life is the proven golden path to health of soul and body as God promises.

"Guard yourself and guard your soul very much" (Deuteronomy 4:9). "The repetition of the word 'guard' alludes to the positive and negative commandments, which protect the limbs and channels which make up the mortal house [the body]. For our rabbis stated (*Zohar, Vayishlach* 170b) that the 248 positive commandments correspond to the 248 limbs of the body, while the 365 prohibitions correspond to the connecting sinews, arteries and channels" (*Kli Yakar* on Deuteronomy 4:9).

Our part

Of all the 613 *mitzvos* that make up the pathway to a healthy life, the *mitzvah* of guarding bodily health has special importance since this is where *we* have to put in effort to properly maintain and protect the instrument with which we perform all the other *mitzvos*. The body is physical and functions according to the natural laws God has fixed. Our part is to provide the body with everything necessary for it to function at its best in accordance with its nature.

As stated by *Rambam*: "A person must avoid anything that may harm the body, and must cultivate healthy habits" (Hilchos Deos 4:1). In other words, the *mitzvah* of self-care has two sides: avoiding all risks to the body and acquiring good health habits.

In the words of the *Shulchan Aruch*, the binding Code of Jewish Law: "It is a positive duty to take all due precautions and avoid anything that may endanger life, as it is written: 'Take care of yourself, and guard your soul'. The sages prohibited many things that involve a risk to life. Anyone who violates such prohibitions, saying 'I'm only putting myself at risk - what business is that of anybody else?' or 'I'm not particular about such things' deserves a lashing, while those who are careful about such things will be blessed" (*Choshen Mishpat* 427, 8-10).

The details of healthy living and care of the body are not in most cases the subject of specific laws. Yet a wealth of wisdom and many different kinds of advice and guidance can be found scattered in passages throughout the Bible, Talmud, Midrash and other rabbinic literature. Outstanding Torah sages knew the importance of healthcare, and saw fit to provide practical guidance in their writings.

Rambam, a giant both in Torah and medicine, devoted an entire chapter at the beginning of the *Mishneh Torah*, his comprehensive compendium of Jewish law, to detailed guidance on proper diet, cleanliness, exercise, sleep and much more (*Hilchos Deos* Chapter 4). *Kitzur Shulchan Aruch*, the Concise Code of Jewish Law, also devotes a whole chapter to the subject (Chapter 32).

The enormous changes in the world in recent generations have caused drastic changes in our whole way of life and even our physical natures and powers of endurance. In contemporary life we cannot always directly apply advice from the classic sources without guidance from present-day experts. Torah law lays down that we must rely on the opinion of expert doctors such as when having to break Shabbos for a dangerously ill person or eating on Yom Kippur. So too we must turn to present-day experts for practical advice about how to maintain health that is faithful to the Torah and applicable in our lives today. In the words of *Kitzur Shulchan Aruch* (32:14): "Every person needs to learn from doctors what are the best foods according to his particular constitution, place and time".

3 Teaching Our Children

"Educate the youth according to his way, even when he grows old, he will not turn from it" (Proverbs 22:6).

How many prayers we pour out to the Almighty for our children. Even before they are born, we beg Him to bring them into the world healthy in soul and body. As soon as they are born, thank G-d, the first thing done in the delivery room is to examine the baby to ascertain that everything is normal and functioning. As our children grow, so do the numbers of details to which we must pay attention to check that everything is developing properly.

We go to enormous lengths for the sake of our children's good and to spare them even the slightest pain and suffering. Every cry, every little sore or sign that indicates that G-d forbid something may not be right arouses immediate anxiety and often sends us running to the doctor.

Are we also prepared to invest effort to save our children from adverse health and future suffering by learning to educate them to guard their health, so that their bodies will serve them well for the good, long years we wish them?

Children are a pledge

As loving parents whose natural need to protectively hold and embrace a child has been fulfilled, we are certainly prepared to invest in the wellbeing of our children. In order to direct this natural feeling in a way that brings maximum benefit to our children, we must always remember that first and foremost these precious children are a pledge entrusted in our hands by the Creator of the World. As G-d's agents, it is our obligation to protect and guard these pledges to the best of our ability. Every Jewish soul that comes into the world adds to the greatness of the Holy One, each one in his or her own unique way. Each boy and girl is a living continuation of the Jewish People. Every single one is an entire world.

An essential part of protecting of these precious pledges is the protection of their health. From earliest childhood we must help them develop healthy habits and instill in them an awareness of the importance of health. What we as parents do to protect our children's health is not enough. As they grow older, we must educate them to take responsibility for their own health, so that when they leave us and embark on their own independent lives, they themselves will take the proper care of themselves.

The *mitzvah* of taking care of our bodies is alluded to in the verse "Guard yourself and guard your soul very much." The continuation of the verse -- "and make them known to your children and your children's children" -- alludes to education!

We are commanded to educate our children in practice of all the *mitzvos*. Our sages also taught us to prepare our children to face the realities of life in this world and the challenges it brings us.

For example, the sages said that a father must teach his son a skill in order for him to make a respectable living. Similarly, they said he must teach his son to swim (*Kiddushin* 29a). Why? In order to save his life if he should ever need it. If our sages instructed us to teach our children skills they might need to save themselves from possible danger, how much more are we obliged to teach them to protect themselves against definite harm from unhealthy practices.

How do you teach children healthcare?

Educating our children to take proper care of their health is a work of many years, often having no set times and applicable in all spheres of life. From birth and in early childhood, the responsibility of caring for children's health falls on their parents, who must provide them with their needs and protect them from hazards. As children grow older, the emphasis shifts to teaching them the importance of health and helping them develop healthy habits.

As soon as children leave the home and enter an educational framework, their teachers must become partners in this enterprise. The nature of the guidance and its content develop according to the needs of each age. Step by step, responsibility for taking care of their health shifts to the children themselves.

In order for the work of education to succeed with the help of G-d, it is necessary to pay careful attention to a number of points:

1. Parents themselves must make every effort to lead a healthy life so as to serve as living examples of what they seek to instill in their children. When parents invest in their children's health, this enhances the quality of life in the home in general.

2. Throughout the day there are constant opportunities to transmit live messages to the children on health: while attending to little children, at mealtimes, around the house, in the classroom, in the street, on a visit to the doctor... It is worth taking advantage of every opportunity. All the different comments and explanations add up, and with time, the message will get through and bring results.

3. Many *mitzvos* are connected with physical functions, from those associated with food and its blessings to saying the blessing *Asher Yatzar*, "Who formed man in wisdom..." An integral part of educating our children to carry out these *mitzvos* is teaching them to satisfy their bodily needs in the manner and within the limitations prescribed by the Torah.

4. Healthy habits are important, but we must avoid turning healthcare into a strict regimen that irritates our children and makes them hate it...

5. We must exercise our imagination to find ways of making healthcare meaningful, practicable and attractive to our children. Everyone needs encouragement. Games, competitions, prizes and other inducements play an important role in gaining children's cooperation in acquiring healthy habits.

An interesting educational method

Once the king's son went mad. He thought he was a turkey. He felt compelled to sit under the table without any clothes on, pulling at bits of bread and bones like a turkey. None of the doctors could do anything to help him or cure him, and they gave up in despair. The king was very sad...

Until a Wise Man came and said, "I can cure him."

What did the Wise Man do? He took off all his clothes, and sat down naked under the table next to the king's son, and also pulled at crumbs and bones.

The Prince asked him, "Who are you and what are you doing here?"

"And what are you doing here?" replied the Wise Man.

"I am a turkey," said the Prince.

"Well I'm also a turkey," said the Wise Man.

The two of them sat there together like this for some time, until they were used to one another.

Then the Wise Man gave a sign, and they threw them shirts. The Wise Man-Turkey said to the king's son, "Do you think a turkey can't wear a shirt? You can wear a shirt and still be a turkey."

The two of them put on shirts.

After a while he gave another sign and they threw them some trousers. Again the Wise Man said, "Do you think if you wear trousers you can't be a turkey?" They put on the trousers.

One by one they put on the rest of their clothes in the same way.

Afterwards, the Wise Man gave a sign and they put down human food from the table. The Wise Man said to the Prince, "Do you think if you eat good food you can't be a turkey anymore? You can eat this food and still be a turkey." They ate.

Then he said to him, "Do you think a turkey has to sit under the table? You can be a turkey and sit up at the table."

This was how the Wise Man dealt with the Prince, until in the end he cured him completely.

-- Rebbe Nachman of Breslov

In the parable of the Prince who thought he was a Turkey, the Prince is a symbol of the rebellious side of children that pushes them not to listen to parents and teachers. Children live in their own world, a world in which the rules and relationships are different from those of adults. We can learn from the Wise Man that it is possible and necessary to give children a feeling of trust that they can do what we ask of them without giving up on their own private world. Similarly, the Wise Man shows us that we can achieve good results only with patience. Getting our children to acquire good health habits is a very important goal. The way to attain it is by going with small steps at their rate. With G-d's help these small steps will lead to great achievements.

4 *Modeh Ani Lefanecha.*
Understanding and appreciating the body

Modeh Ani - **"I thank You, living, enduring King, for You have returned my soul within me in kindness, great is Your faithfulness."**

These are the words with which the Jew begins each day on opening his eyes after his night-time sleep. "Thank You!"

One of the main reasons for our daily recital of these words and the ensuing morning blessings is to develop and strengthen our gratitude to G-d, Who created us, soul and body, crowning glory of the creation! With endless love and kindness, He provides us with all our needs each day and watches over every limb of our bodies at every moment. This is not something we may take for granted.

Our Sages understood human nature, and they knew that people do tend to take daily occurrences for granted, no matter how wonderful they may be. For this reason the rabbis instituted that we should start our day by devoting some time to reflection upon G-d's kindnesses to us while reciting *Modeh Ani* followed by *Asher Yatzar*, "Who formed man.", the blessing over our bodily functioning, *Pokeach Ivrim*, "Who gives sight to the blind", *Matir Asurim*, "Who releases the bound, *Zokef Kefufim*, "Who straightens those who are bent over" and the other morning blessings. Each day we should strive to say these words with renewed gratitude.

Awareness of the wonder of bodily functioning strengthens our motivation to take proper care of our bodies in accordance with G-d's commandment. The more we recognize and understand the body's amazing powers, the more carefully we will guard and maintain the precious gift of health. The better care we take of our bodies, the better our bodies will serve us in our service of G-d.

Getting to know the body

How can we teach our children appreciation and thankfulness for the wonderful body G-d has given them, in order to bring them to take proper care of themselves?

Every age and stage in the development of children calls for its own approach to this aspect of their education. Each boy and girl is a unique world. Parents must be sensitive to the special nature of each child in guiding him or her to develop an appreciation of the body and a sense of thankfulness to G-d for His kindness. Small children can obviously not be expected to attain a mature grasp of bodily functioning. Even as children grow older, their interest in what is important to adults is often limited. Nevertheless, at these critical stages in their lives, when they are beginning to learn about their bodies, there are many opportunities to develop their awareness of the wonders of bodily functioning and their sense of gratitude to the Maker of the World for His constant kindness to us.

Educating our children begins long before they enter an educational framework outside the house, even before they begin to speak. A baby sucking his mother's milk already hears her speaking to him. The very words and expressions we use when tending little children are part of their education. The baby starts to know his name. He is conscious of different tones of voice and different kinds of feelings, positive and negative. Soon, the baby starts reacting with a smile or by crying, reactions that indicate a level of understanding.

As parents it is natural for us to want to teach and enrich our children as much as possible, even when they are babies. Soon after a baby says his first words - "Mama", "Dada" - we usually start playfully teaching him or her the names of the different parts of the body, "Hand", "Mouth", "Nose", "Eye", "Ear". With the right facial expressions and tone of voice, these little games convey to the small child the message that this or that part of his or her body is good, important, precious.

As children develop physically, mentally and spiritually, the scope for teaching them about the beauty and wisdom of the way our bodies function widens, whether at mealtimes, when washing and changing them, putting them to bed, playing with them and other shared times, through games, stories, songs. Children themselves are often naturally interested in certain aspects of their bodies, like why they have to eat, and why we breathe. It is good to try to arouse children's interest in the subject, such as by pointing out the wonder of being able to lift, give or take with the hand, run and jump with the feet. Children's questions and responses are normally the best guide to what we can communicate at any given stage and how.

Enhancing our children's awareness of the wonders of their bodies and thankfulness for them is not separable from the education we must give them in each of the specific areas of healthcare, such as cleanliness and hygiene, safety, proper diet, movement and exercise. This awareness should be an integral part of the teaching and guidance we give them in each area.

For example, in the familiar case of the little child who comes running to Mummy with a scratch crying that he's been "cut", we can soothe the child and even "heal" the "cut" with words. As we put on a plaster, we can calm the child by telling him, "It could have been much more serious, and Baruch HaShem it's only a scratch." and, "Let's pray to HaShem to heal it. BeEzras HaShem it will soon get better." With an extra kiss, the boy runs off happy and content.

In the area of hygiene and cleanliness, one of the early stages in children's education is toilet training. Part of this is explaining to the child that it is necessary to go to the toilet when he or she feels the need, and that this is a mitzvah. According to the child's level of understanding, we can explain that G-d created our body's way of digesting food in the stomach and intestines so that it takes out the good from our food, absorbing it in our bodies, while expelling the waste in the food, which would otherwise be harmful to the body. Our part is that we must go to the toilet when we feel the need in order to help our body clean itself.

When teaching our children to appreciate and take proper care for their bodies, it is unnecessary to enter into detailed explanations of the different body parts, especially not those that are of no relevance to children. What is important is to provide our children with a basic practical understanding of the main body parts and systems relating to areas where they have a role to play in caring for their health. These include digestion and elimination, which relate to proper nutrition, cleanliness and hygiene, blood circulation and breathing, bones, joints and muscles, which relate to proper movement, exercise and avoidance of injury, and so on. The goal is to teach the children what they need to know about these aspects of the body so that they will understand the importance of taking proper care in each area.

As a general rule, when we seek to teach our children healthy habits of self-care, physical and mental, we must make sure that the words and concepts we use express the Torah view of man and his body as the work of the hands of G-d. He watches over us every day and every moment, and He wants us to play our part and do what is necessary to take proper care of ourselves: "And take good care of your souls".

The blessing of Asher Yatzar

Several times every day we have an opportunity to express our gratitude to G-d for the wonderful working of our body when we say the blessing *Asher Yatzar* after relieving ourselves. *Asher Yatzar* is the blessing that our Sages instituted over the wisdom in the design of man's body and the wonders of its functioning. After relieving ourselves, cleaning our bodies and washing our hands, we must pause for a moment from all our activities and focus exclusively on saying the blessing, reflecting on G-d's wonders and expressing our gratitude for them.

A number of sources mention that recital of the blessing of *Asher Yatzar* with attention to its meaning is itself conducive to good health. When a person is aware of and appreciates the kindness someone does him, the benefactor is happy to shower him with even more kindness. How much more so will G-d, whose goodness is unending, increase His goodness and kindness to us if we truly appreciate them.

Often people begin to appreciate health more when, G-d forbid, it is lacking, forcing them to pray and expend great effort in trying to restore it. It is better to invest in expressing thanks in *Asher Yatzar for* what G-d has already given us rather than to have to ask for it back if G-d forbid we lose it. In *Asher Yatzar* our Sages provided us with a beautiful way of expressing our thanks to G-d for the wonderful body He has given us.

Teaching children to say Asher Yatzar

Asher Yatzar is one of the first blessings with which we open our day. It is also among the first blessings that children learn. At this stage teachers enter as partners with the parents in the work of educating the children. At first the children are taught to recite the blessing at the start of each day. Later on they are taught to recite the blessing each time they attend to their needs after washing their hands.

As part of the education of the children in awareness of the wonders of the body and gratitude for G-d's kindness, it is necessary to explain clearly the simple meaning of *Asher Yatzar* and the great importance of saying it properly. We need to use our imagination to vividly communicate the wonder of the body's different parts and functioning, digestion, circulation and breathing, vision, hearing, smell, taste, touch. Not only must we arouse the children's interest in the amazing wonder of the body. We must also teach them Who created it, and that they must give expression to their gratitude in the blessing of *Asher Yatzar.*

Young children are not expected to understand the deep meaning of the blessing and to recite it with full attention every time. Nevertheless, it is good to habituate them from an early age to enunciate the words of the blessing properly. Parents need to emphasize repeatedly the importance of giving proper attention to saying *Asher Yatzar* so that it should not become a matter of thoughtless repetition. It can help to encourage children with special campaigns, competitions, prizes and the like. In many homes an attractively printed version of *Asher Yatzar* is hung above the wash basin outside the restroom.

May we and our children always be able to recite *Asher Yatzar* in thanks to G-d that our bodies are healthy!

5 Cleanliness and Hygiene

Rabbi Akiva said: "Once I followed Rabbi Yehoshua into the restroom and I learned three things from him." Ben Azai said to Rabbi Akiva, "How could you be so bold with your teacher?" Rabbi Akiva replied: "It is Torah, and I need to learn!" (*Berachos* 62a).

Teaching our children about cleanliness begins practically from the moment they are born. We go to great efforts to keep our children clean, and also to separate them from what is spiritually impure. Not only do we wash and bath them and change their diapers. We also wash even little children's hands with *Negelwasser* when they wake up from their night's sleep in order to remove *Tum'ah*, the unclean night-time spirit. Not only do we teach our children to use the toilet and clean themselves properly. We also train them to wash their hands on leaving the bathroom and the like, and also before prayer and Torah study. We teach them to clean and wash their hands very well before touching food. We also teach them *Netilas Yadayim*, ritual washing of the hands before eating bread.

The message we are giving our children is that we must keep ourselves clean, and also, we must keep ourselves pure. Physical cleanliness and spiritual purity are two different sides of cleanliness. Both are bound up with each other. The Torah teaches us to clean our bodies of their waste products and to dispose of them properly. The purpose is to keep ourselves and our surroundings clean. Only then can G-d's spirit dwell among us: "Your camp must be holy" (Deuteronomy 23:15).

The cleanliness of our bodies and surroundings is one of the principal foundations of purity. We are not allowed to say words of prayer or Torah when our bodies are not clean or in a place that is not clean. Not only does physical cleanliness contribute to our general sense of well-being. Physical cleanliness is essential for good health. The body can only function properly when it cleanses itself of its various waste products. We must play our part in the cleansing process with proper habits of toilet, washing and general cleanliness.

Waste and dirt are the breeding grounds of harmful microbes that cause infections and illness. To avoid harm and illness, we are obliged to follow the rules of cleanliness and hygiene. This is part of the commandment, "Take care of your souls". Then our bodies will be a fit vessel fit to carry out G-d's laws and a worthy sanctuary for the soul.

Teaching children about cleanliness and hygiene

There are no fixed rules about when to start training children in proper habits of hygiene and cleanliness. Most parents have an intuitive understanding of their children, and will know when to start and how to guide each child in accordance with his or her age, character and level of development.

The first step

The obvious first practical step is when we start teaching children to use the toilet and everything that goes with this. This is usually around the age of two or three, sometimes earlier, sometimes later. Training a child may take anywhere between four or five weeks to six months or more. Parents seeking guidance in toilet-training a child can turn to others who already have experience or to a doctor.

In the first stages of teaching a child to use the toilet, each time the child needs to go, the parent (or home help, nursery teacher, etc) goes with the child to help him. This is the time to start teaching the child in his language and according to his level of understanding that dirt and waste are not good for us and we must remove them from our bodies and flush them away. For this very reason, we must not hold back when we need to attend to our needs. As soon as we feel the need, we should go as soon as possible.

We must teach the child to clean himself properly, and then wash his hands thoroughly with soap and water. The next step is to encourage the child to manage independently in the restroom without needing help, being sure to practice the rules of cleanliness and hygiene that he has learned.

Washing hands

Washing our hands after our night-time sleep, before prayer, before eating bread, after attending to our bodily needs and on other occasions is an integral part of the daily life of the Jew. Our children need to learn that having *clean* hands and having *pure* hands are two things that are bound together. We teach them that there is an obligation to wash their hands before bread (*Netilas Yadayim*). It is also important to teach them that their hands must be *clean*. Washing our hands in order to clean them does not exempt us from *Netilas Yadayim*. So too, *Netilas Yadayim* does not exempt us from first making sure that our hands are clean!

As children grow older and become more understanding, we should explain to them why we must keep our hands clean. We carry millions of tiny microbes on our hands. Most are not harmful, but some can cause infections, diarrhea, parasites, flu and even more serious illnesses. Harmful microbes can pass onto our bodies from contact with dirt in the toilet, dirty towels, door handles, stair-rails and the like handled by people carrying infectious microbes. If we touch our mouths, nose, ears, eyes or an open cut or wound with dirty hands, these microbes can enter inside our bodies. Thorough washing of the hands greatly reduces the risk of infection by these microbes.

Children should be taught to wash their hands carefully

AFTER

1. Leaving the toilet or bathroom

2. Touching garbage and anything dirty (including children's play-sand).

3. Touching a dirty nose

4. Touching an open cut or sore

5. Touching an animal, bird or insect

6. Touching raw meat or fish

BEFORE

1. Touching food

2. Eating

3. Tending a cut or sore

4. Inserting or removing contact lenses

The hands should be washed with soap and water. When hot water is not available, the hands should be washed thoroughly with cold water and soap. The entire surface of the hand should be washed up to the wrist, including the palms and back of the hands, the fingers and under the nails. The hands should be rubbed together with soap and rinsed well with water. The hands should be dried with a clean towel, preferably disposable, or with a hand-drying machine.

Factors that contribute to better standards of hygiene and cleanliness include:

1. Adequate supplies of toilet paper

2. Soap for washing of hands

3. Clean towels. Where possible in educational and other institutions, these should be disposable, or hand-drying machines should be provided.

4. It is best to keep children's nails short, and they should be taught the importance of keeping them clean.

5. Parents should provide their children with tissues to clean their noses.

6. Parents and teachers must repeatedly remind children about the importance of keeping their hands clean in order to make sure that the message gets across.

Washing the body

"The one who tends to his soul is the man of kindness" (Proverbs 11:17). This verse applies to Hillel the Elder! When he used to leave his students and go on his way, they would accompany him and ask: "Rabbi, where are you going?" "To carry out and do a mitzvah," he would reply. "Which mitzvah is that?" "To wash in the bath-house." "Why?" they would ask. "Is it a mitzvah to wash?" "Yes," he replied. "The statues of kings that stand in public theaters and circuses have a special officer whose job is to rinse and scrub them to keep them clean. They pay him for this, and he sits with the elite of the kingdom. How much more so must I wash and clean myself. For I am made in the form and likeness of the King of kings, as it is written "For He made man in the likeness of G-d" (Genesis 9:6; Vayikra Rabbah 34:3).

When parents take care to keep their children clean from the earliest age, consciousness of cleanliness and its importance penetrates deep inside the children. Everything parents do to keep their little children clean, rinse their hands and faces, wash and bath them, is a part of helping them acquire clean habits. As they grow older, we should explain to them according to their understanding why it is so important for them to keep their bodies clean. This way they will come to do so of their own accord.

We should explain to our children in addition to the good feeling when we are clean, first and foremost we are thereby guarding our health. The skin is one of the most important body parts, even though many people don't pay too much attention to it unless there is a problem. The protective coat with which G-d in His wisdom has our bodies not only protects us from harm from the world around us. Our skin also plays an important role in the elimination of certain bodily waste products. Our task is to wash and clean our skin to keep it healthy.

Water has an essential role in keeping the body clean, and we should teach our children to wash regularly. The frequency with which one needs to wash varies from person to person depending on individual physical factors, daily activity, environment, the weather and other factors. Just as it is no good to wash too little, so there is no need to exaggerate.

It is best to wash the body in warm water using a delicate soap. An important part of washing is thorough rinsing of all traces of soap in order to avoid irritation. Children should be taught to dry themselves well after washing.

Regular washing of the hair is an important part of overall bodily cleanliness. Having clean, orderly hair gives a good feeling and contributes to a pleasing appearance. When children's hair is clean and healthy, this also helps against the "Third Plague" - lice.

Clean nails are also an important part of bodily cleanliness. Parents should cut their children's nails, hands and feet, before they grow too long. It is good to teach children that cutting nails is one of the things we do each week prior to and in preparation for Shabbos. Any time that dirt gathers under the fingernails, they should be brushed with soap and water. It is worth teaching children how to cut the nails of their big toe in such a way as to avoid ingrowing toenails.

Even though the specific obligation is only to wash the hands [each morning], nevertheless it is a mitzvah also to wash ones face, for "G-d made everything for His sake" (Proverbs 16:4). The body is created to serve G-d and is the garment of the soul - and "man's soul is G-d's lamp" (ibid. 20:27). It is proper to show respect for the garment in the same way as a king's officers take good care to keep the garments they receive from the king free of all dirt. In the same way, it is proper to wash one's face and keep it clean. Similarly, the clothes a person wears - and this applies particularly to a Torah scholar - should be kept clean and free of all dirt.

Chayey Adam 2:6

Cleanliness in puberty

Puberty is a new stage in development that parents must be aware of. As children enter this important time in their lives, parents should draw their attention to the need to take extra care to keep clean because of the physical changes in their bodies. The skin and hair are likely to become more oily. The sweat glands are more active not only when we are hot, but also as a reaction to feelings and emotions. The armpits, folds of the body, palms of the hands and soles of the feet exude a more concentrated sweat that may cause unpleasant odors.

Adolescents should be encouraged to pay greater attention to bodily cleanliness and orderly appearance, and to bath or shower, change their clothes, have their hair cut, cut their nails and so on as necessary. Where body odor is a problem, a deodorant may help. In cases of excessive sweating, consult a doctor.

One of the most widespread and troublesome problems of puberty is acne. The first step in treating acne is to keep the face clean and to wash it with tepid water a couple of times of day. Do not touch the infected areas. If the problem is particularly troublesome a doctor can recommend suitable treatment.

A Clean Mouth

Keeping the body clean applies not only to the exterior but also to the interior. Cleanliness of the mouth is of primary importance, since the mouth is one of the main channels through which microbes can enter the body. The dangers are particularly serious in the case of small children, whose understanding of what is good for them and what can harm them is still limited.

Little children have little or no sense of the boundaries they must maintain in their interaction with the environment. They do not distinguish between what they may touch and what is dangerous, what they may put in their mouths and what can harm them. Little children naturally tend to put everything they find in their mouths - their fingers, toys, and then, when they begin to crawl, whatever they find on the floor, including pieces of food, buttons, pins and worse.

As parents who want to keep our children from danger at any price, we must constantly watch them to see that they do not put anything harmful in their mouths. There are some things that everyone knows to be dangerous, but there are other hazards that not everyone is aware of:

1. Food and candies that have fallen on the floor are dirty and should not be put in the mouth unless they can be washed properly.

2. Anything that has touched one person's mouth should not be put in someone else's mouth. Food, candies, drinking bottles etc. should not be passed from mouth to mouth.

3. Children have a tendency to touch their shoes, socks, feet, head, dirty nose and worse. They must learn not to put their hands in their mouth or touch food without first washing their hands.

> The sages prohibited eating and drinking anything that most people would find disgusting... They also prohibited eating with dirty hands and on dirty utensils, for all these things come under the rule, "Do not make your souls loathsome." Everyone who is careful in these matters brings extra holiness and purity to his soul and cleanses his soul in honor of the Holy One blessed be He, as it is said, "And you shall sanctify yourselves and be holy, for I am holy" (Leviticus 11:44).
>
> Rambam, Hilchos Maachalos Asuros (Forbidden Foods) 17:29-32

Care of teeth

Healthy teeth are an important part of bodily health. Healthy teeth enable us to chew our food well, which is the start of good digestion. Good teeth also help us speak clearly as well as contributing to a pleasing appearance.

The effort which parents put into keeping their children's teeth healthy and teaching them to take proper care of them is a sound investment that can save a lot of suffering and heavy expenses later on. One of the main causes of tooth decay today is the high quantity of sugar in the average daily diet. When remains of our food stay in the mouth for extended periods, a thin layer of sugars (plaque) forms on the teeth, which encourages increased activity by bacteria, leading to tooth decay, cavities, infections, retreating gums and severe pain. Keeping the mouth and the teeth clean, especially after eating, is the main way to avoid these problems.

Parents should pay attention to their children's teeth from the moment they begin to sprout and perhaps even before. Some parents clean their child's gums with a soft, damp cloth after meals even before their teeth appear. Unfortunately, parents sometimes bear a heavy share of responsibility for severe teeth problems among children. For some reason, many feel obliged to feed their child with a bottle whose contents are usually sweetened. The bottle remains in the child's mouth for long periods, and not infrequently, the child falls asleep with the bottle in his mouth. Extended contact of the teeth with the sugars in the food causes increased bacterial activity that can cause "bottle caries", deformation and premature falling of the milk teeth, and poor development of second teeth. Long before we start teaching our children to keep their teeth clean, we should do what we can to make sure their teeth are healthy in the first place!

Brushing the teeth

The first habit to teach our children to care for their teeth is regular cleaning. In order to instill this habit, it is good to early, even from the age of two or three, though initially the gains in cleanliness may be limited. To encourage the child, one can purchase a soft toothbrush and "tasty" children's toothpaste. Later on, it is worthwhile to take the child for a dental examination - hopefully before he has any pain in his teeth. Thank G-d today there are dentists who specialize in treating children and are sensitive to their needs. The dentist (or assistant) will explain to the child the importance of cleaning our teeth and give him a practical demonstration.

Children should be taught to clean their teeth at least twice a day, in the morning and especially before they go to sleep at night. They should be taught that whenever possible, it is good to rinse their mouths with water after each meal, and especially after eating sweets.

Parents should reinforce the dentist's message by giving their children practical training in how to brush their teeth. Every tooth has three exposed surfaces - outside, inside and top. One should systematically brush all the teeth in each jaw, the upper and the lower, those in front and those at the sides and back, on the right and on the left. Brushing the teeth should continue for about three minutes. One should teach children that the purpose is not so much to polish as to clean the teeth, as well as to clean between them and where they are attached to the gums.

Caring for children's teeth is a constant process in which both parents and children have a share: The parents' part is to make sure the children play their part by regularly brushing their teeth! Parents must find ways of encouraging their children to take proper care of teeth, such as with prizes - as long as they aren't sweets! A dental examination is recommended twice a year.

6. Danger! Take Care

Wherever there is a potentially life-endangering pitfall or obstacle, it is a positive commandment to remove it, to be on guard against it and to take very good care in the matter, as the Torah says: "Guard yourself and guard your soul." (Deuteronomy 4:9-10). And if one leaves dangerous pitfalls and obstacles and fails to remove them, he has not fulfilled the positive commandment, while also transgressing the negative commandment of "Do not put blood upon your house" (Deuteronomy 22:8). The Sages prohibited many things that can endanger life... Anyone who violates these and similar prohibitions, saying "What business is it of others if I choose to put myself in danger" or "I am not bothered about such things" is liable to get lashes for rebellion against the Sages, while those who are careful will be blessed with good.

(*Shulchan Aruch, Choshen Mishpat* 427: 8-10).

The Torah obliges us to protect ourselves from dangers and to keep them well away. Today more than ever we have many occasions to keep these two mitzvahs of "Guard yourself" (the positive mitzvah) and "Do not put blood." (the negative). There have always been dangers, and it was always necessary to take care. But the wonders of modern science and technology have brought many new dangers inside our homes, on the street and everywhere else.

It is not enough to be aware of dangers. It is our duty to do everything possible to protect ourselves from them. The rule that "a danger is more serious than a ritual prohibition" (*Chulin 10a*) applies to the two mitzvahs of "Guard yourself" and "Do not put blood". In other words, negligence in the face of danger is more serious than violating Torah prohibitions such as against forbidden foods. Certainly, "We may not rely on miracles" (*Pesachim* 64b).

Teaching safety to children

As soon as children are born, the responsibility for their safety falls upon the parents. A baby obviously cannot take care of himself, and we the parents have to keep our eyes open all hours of the day. We watch our babies in the crib, the stroller and even when they're in our arms.

The need to supervise a child grows the more active he becomes, especially the moment he starts crawling and walking. Now he can get all over the place. Our houses are likely to have plenty of electrical sockets and appliances, fragile items, sharp knives and tools, strong cleaning materials and other sources of danger. It is not enough to keep the child away from danger. His growing independence makes it vital that we try to start teaching him what he may touch and what he must not touch, where he may play and what he must keep away from in the kitchen, the bathroom, on the balcony and everywhere else in the house. As soon as the child starts going out of the house to explore the wider world, we must correspondingly expand the scope of what we teaching him to include the stairway, the yard, the playground, the roads...

Parents normally have an instinctive understanding of their children and how to find the right language, tone of voice, facial expressions and appropriate gestures to communicate the necessary message to each child. At every age, safety education must be in accordance with the development and understanding of the child. Our warnings and explanations must be very clear and are most effective when we give vivid examples of what can happen by ignoring danger.

Some important points to remember:

1. We must be consistent about what we allow our children to do and what we do not allow them to do. This way they will not be confused, and they won't come to think we are joking with them.

2. Safety warnings usually need to be repeated often on different occasions in order to penetrate children's consciousness with the correct message and turn safety into a habit.

3. Most important, we must never take chances and rely on children to take proper care even after giving them precise instructions. We must carry on supervising them! Even after warning them repeatedly about a certain danger, we cannot take it for granted that they understand the real meaning of the danger.

Children's safety education is an extended process. As they grow older and become more independent, our ability to supervise them is more limited. It is our duty to educate and prepare them well for the stage when we are not at hand to take care of them, so they will G-d willing be able to guard and protect themselves from danger.

We must also help them develop a deep sense of responsibility so that they will not endanger *others*. Likewise we must teach them that at times others are liable to act in ways that endanger *them*, whether through irresponsibility, lack of caution or for any other reason. They must be aware of this and learn to take appropriate precautions, such as in the playground, when crossing the road, and so on.

Accidents can happen anywhere and at any time. With G-d's help it is in our power to prevent many accidents if we are aware of the things that are likely to cause them. Parents must learn to recognize possible dangers to which their children are likely to be exposed. This way the parents can take the necessary precautions to protect their children as well as teaching them to protect themselves.

Taking proper care of our children includes acquiring a basic knowledge of first aid in the event of an accident in the home. Every home should have a first aid kit. Parents should also teach their children fundamentals such as the need to keep a cut clean, what to do in the event of a small burn, insect bite, etc. An organization to teach children first aid basics would be a blessed enterprise!

Parents should also certify that their children's school or Talmud Torah also has first aid facilities and someone who knows how to give first aid, and when to call a doctor or send a case to hospital.

We must always remember that whatever we do to protect ourselves from danger is fulfillment of a positive mitzvah of the Torah. We are trying to do our part to carry out G-d's will in the faith that G-d in His kindness will watch over us and protect us always.

Safety in the home

Studies indicate that the majority of home accidents involve electricity, fire, water, poisonous substances or falls. The more aware we are of the various causes of accidents, the more we can avoid them.

Electricity

There must be a rule that "Children do not touch sockets". Parents must ensure that sockets not in use are covered, preferably with childproof covers. Do not leave sockets that have become detached from the wall, or exposed wires. It is dangerous to leave long electrical or phone wires trailing across the floor.

As far as possible, electrical appliances should be kept out of children's reach. When this is impossible, we must make it clear to the children that they are not allowed to touch them. In teaching children about the dangers of electricity, parents should put particular emphasis on the serious danger if water comes in contact with electrical sockets, wires and appliances. Together with the explanations, parents must continue carefully supervising their children.

It is desirable to install an electrical safety switch that automatically shuts off the electricity supply when an appliance is faulty or in contact with water, etc.

It is desirable to contact licensed electricians for the installation of an electrical safety switch that will automatically shut off the electrical supply when an appliance is faulty or in contact with water, etc.

Fire

We must take special precautions and do everything possible to avoid anything that might lead to a fire in the home. Too many appliances should not be attached to a single outlet. An appliance that emits a bad smell or smoke should be turned off immediately. Lamps, heaters and other appliances must be kept away from bedding, curtains and other fabrics. Some synthetic fabrics are particularly flammable and must be kept well away from flames. Fire and electrical heaters must be properly covered with safety-grilles and children must be warned not to come near them or to stick anything into the heater.

A burning fire (food cooking on the stove, lighted candles) should not be left without supervision. Thank G-d, as Jews we have many opportunities to light candles in our homes on Shabbos, festivals and other occasions. We must see that the candles are always well out or children's reach, and we must warn our children not to come near fire, and even then, we must keep careful watch over them. Special care must be taken when lighting candles in the Succah.

Many children are fascinated by fire, and there are some children who despite their fear will not pass up an opportunity to play with fire. We must warn children again and again that fire can cause a terrible disaster. Children must not be left unsupervised near a fire or flame of any kind, nor should children have access to matches and lighters, etc. Special supervision of children is necessary when lighting bonfires on Lag BaOmer, burning Chametz before Pesach or having a "Kumzitz" or barbecue. At Purim time children should not be allowed to play with dangerous fireworks, fire crackers and the like.

Water

Cases of children drowning in water in the home are all too common, and we must take extra precautions to avoid such accidents. When little children are around, it is dangerous to leave buckets of water around in the bathroom etc. unless the children are properly supervised, as they must be when playing in a tub or pool of water. Even when the water is very shallow, there is always the danger that a small child may fall with his face in the water. There is also a danger that a child may fall head first into the toilet or bath. The doors of the toilet and bathroom should be kept closed to prevent children entering. Small children must not be left in the bath unsupervised if there is the possibility that they could open a hot tap. One should always check the temperature of the bath or shower before putting a child in the water. Likewise the temperature of the child's bottle must be checked before feeding.

Poisonous and other dangerous substances

All cleaning fluids, medicines, alcohol, paint, pest control substances and all other poisonous and dangerous substances must be kept out of reach of children and where possible locked away. Children must be warned repeatedly not to touch these substances, let alone putting them in their mouths.

Plastic bags are made of materials through which it is impossible to breathe. Children have a tendency to play with plastic bags and sometimes put them over their heads, which can cause suffocation. Plastic bags should be kept out of reach of children, and they must be taught never to put a plastic bag over their faces or heads.

Slipping and falling

Little children generally have little awareness of danger. We must teach them that it can be dangerous to climb on furniture or anything else that is not stable, and that if they have climbed somewhere and cannot get down, it is best to ask for help and not to jump. At the same time, parents should do what they can around the house to minimize the possibility of children's slipping, falling and getting hurt.

When applying "polish" to the floor, one should choose a non-slip product. Especially when children are around, a polished floor should not be covered with rugs and carpets that might cause them to slip or trip. All obstacles should be removed from passageways, stairs and the like. Corners of items of furniture (tables, beds), marble kitchen surfaces, etc. should be rounded or padded to avoid injuries. Proper lighting helps avoid accidents.

Those who live on upper floors should see that windows have proper safety bars and that the railings around balconies and roofs are high enough and strong enough. Children must be taught never to climb on chairs or anything else near the railings. As soon as a child is old enough to crawl around the house, the door leading to the stairs must be kept closed. Duplex homes should have safety-gates at the top and bottom of the stairs.

In the kitchen

Small children and especially crawling babies should as far as possible be kept well away from the stove and oven. Check that the buttons controlling the flow of gas are shut when not in use. If there is a smell of gas, try to check the source. If there is a leak, close the safety tap and call a technician as soon as possible. When lighting the gas, a lighter with a long handle is preferable to matches.

When cooking with pots that have long handles,

the pots should be arranged on the stove so that the handles do not stick out so that there is no danger of catching on them when passing by and pulling them over. Some stoves have a guard that prevents pots from moving or slipping out of place. When baking, be sure to keep children well away from the oven before opening the door.

Utensils containing hot food and liquids should not be left within reach of children. Nor should they be left on a table if there is any possibility that a child could pull at the tablecloth.

Knives, scissors and other sharp utensils must be kept out of small children's reach, and the same applies to tools. Electrical appliances that are not in use should be disconnected and the outlet covered. Strong or poisonous substances should not be stored in the kitchen. The garbage bin should be kept covered.

In the bathroom

It is best to keep electrical outlets and switches out of the bathroom itself to avoid the possibility of contact with water. If there is an electrical heater in the bathroom, it must be mounted high up on the wall. Any electrical switches and outlets in the bathroom must be out of children's reach. When bathing or showering, any electrical appliance that could possibly come in contact with water should be turned off.

It is advisable to attach non-skid strips to the bottom of the bath to prevent slipping. As elsewhere in the home, sharp instruments and strong or poisonous substances in the bathroom should be kept well out of reach of children.

The bedroom

Choose only a safe method of heating the children's room, such as a radiator that has no exposed fire and cannot emit dangerous gases. In any event, the heater and all other electrical appliances must be kept well away from curtains, bedding and other fabrics.

A child's crib should have side-rails that are sufficiently high to prevent any possibility that the child might climb out and fall. Crib slats should not be too wide apart so that the child will not be able to push his head in between and get caught. Soft pillows and bedding and anything else that could suffocate the baby must be removed. Ribbons, strings, straps and anything else that could cause strangulation must be kept well out of the child's reach.

As a general rule, toys for children of all ages should be chosen with an eye for their safety. Toys for babies should not be breakable or easily torn and should not have attachments that can be pulled off. Small toys should be kept well away from babies as they can put them in the mouth and swallow them. Make sure that all toys and other products for use with babies and children should meet the necessary official safety standards.

Safety outside

As children start to go outside the house, they become exposed to many new dangers - in the street, the playground and everywhere else. Children's ability to estimate dangers and their seriousness is usually limited. When small children are outside they must be under constant supervision. The older and more independent they become, it is our parental duty to teach them about common dangers and how to guard against them. As soon as children enter an educational framework, the teachers and educators must take their share in supervising the children, and they too must train and guide the children in their care to take care and avoid danger.

In the playground

Playing outside is an important and healthy activity that greatly contributes to children's development. The more they grow, the more they use their bodies to run, jump, climb. We should give them every encouragement, as this is how they gain strength and develop their coordination and other skills and abilities. At the same time, we need to watch over them to ensure that they do not put themselves in danger or endanger others. We should teach them to use playground equipment properly, not to push other children, and to watch how and where they are jumping and running.

Not only must we teach children to play carefully and avoid danger in the playground. It is also most important to help them develop a responsible attitude towards what belongs to others, and especially towards public property. Children benefit from the playground and the equipment: it is forbidden to destroy them!

Similarly, children should be taught not to throw litter and to take care to keep public places clean just as we keep our homes clean.

Exposure to the sun

"A sun of righteousness with healing in its wings" (Malachi 3:20). The rays of the sun have healing qualities. At the same time, excessive exposure to the sun can cause serious damage to the skin and even cancer. Too much sun can also cause dehydration and sunstroke. Parents must keep children from exposure to the sun on hot days and especially during the hottest hours of the day. When children go out into the open they should be equipped with suitable clothing and sun hats as well as sufficient drink.

Safety on the roads

"All roads are likely to be places of danger" (*Yerushalmi Berachos* 4, 4).

Our Sages' rule that all roads must be considered dangerous is more applicable today than at any other time. Accidents are one of the leading causes of death and injury in the world. Parents must repeat to their children over and over again, from the earliest age, that the road is a very dangerous place. When parents have occasion to take their children on the street, where they see cars, traffic lights, pedestrian crossings and so on, this is a good time to give children practical education in safety precautions on the streets and roads and dangers they must be aware of.

Even after teaching children the rules of road safety, we must be certain they follow them in practice before we allow them to cross the road alone. This rule certainly applies to parents who allow their children to ride on bicycles. Never take risks!

The main rules we must repeatedly instill in children are:

1. Any place where there are moving cars is a place of possible danger.

2. It is forbidden to run out into the road.

3. The sidewalk is not a place to play, and certainly not the road.

4. Cross the road only at a green light or pedestrian crossing. Small children who have to cross the road should ask help from an adult.

5. When children step down from the school bus, they must immediately move onto the sidewalk and wait until the school bus moves off and drives away. Never stand in front of or behind a car as the driver may drive the car forwards or backwards without seeing the child.

6. While teaching our children all the necessary safety precautions on the streets and roads, we must also instill them with a deep awareness that the first step on leaving the house to go out must be to turn to the Creator of the World to ask His protection from all danger.

When the children enter an educational framework, parents must work in conjunction with their children's teachers to see that the children are thoroughly trained in all aspects of road safety, with regular reviews of all the main rules. Today's leading rabbis have given their full support and encouragement to this endeavor. Responsibility for children's education in road safety lies not only with parents and teachers but also with adult pedestrians and drivers in general. When adults serve as living examples of proper care on the roads, children will learn from them and follow their example, thereby avoiding many accidents.

Caution with strangers

On today's streets it is not only the cars that are dangerous. There are also dangerous people, and children should be taught basic rules of caution:

1. Small children must not talk to strangers or take something from them. They must not go off in their company and certainly never get into a stranger's car. Children should be taught to keep well away from strangers. They should be taught that if a stranger should ever take hold of them and try to take them, they should do everything in their power to get away. They should have no shame about shouting and screaming and making as much noise as possible in order to attract someone's attention.

2. In the event of a suspicious object, children should be taught to keep well away and to call an adult for help. It is desirable to teach children not to pick up toys or other objects thrown in the street.

Smoking

Many of the hazards we have discussed so far pose an immediate danger to our children and are likely to encounter every day in the house and outside. Parents of small children may consider smoking a remote problem - and so may it always remain. But the truth is that smoking is not such a far-off risk. Children are often exposed to smokers and cigarette smoke. Unfortunately, our children often see adults smoking, and among them, people they are taught to respect. This may encourage them to think smoking is not such a serious problem.

The dangers of smoking and its results have been known for years. Smoking causes damage to the lungs and heart and general health. Not only is smoking a waste of precious money, it also causes an unpleasant odor on the smoker's mouth and clothes and gives his teeth and hands an unsightly appearance. Recent research proves beyond all doubt that the harm caused by inhaling other people's cigarette smoke ("passive smoking") is as great as the harm caused to the smokers themselves.

Doctors are unanimously opposed to smoking. In all advanced countries, health regulations require that cigarette packs must carry a warning that smoking is dangerous to health. Yet in spite of everything, smoking is very widespread. Every year the ranks of smokers are swelled by tens of thousands of new smokers, most of them young. The mere sight of adults smoking encourages many young people (and even children) to start smoking, some out of curiosity, others because of a desire to assert their independence, to show how old they are or make an impression on their peers, or as a sign of rebellion. Unfortunately, Purim has turned into a time for children to try smoking, and from there it's often a short road to regular smoking.

Education against smoking should start from a young age. Just as we inoculate small children against dangerous diseases, so we should find ways to "immunize" our children against the temptation to smoke long before they are exposed to it. When parents are with their children and come across people who are smoking, this can be an opportunity to explain to the children that this is not a good habit and that smoking damages people's health. Some parents specify the damage that can be caused by smoking in detail in order to foster an aversion for the habit in their children.

As a general rule, children must understand that

their parents are clear and unwavering in their opposition to smoking as well as to alcohol consumption and all other forms of substance abuse. At the same time, parents must be open and willing to answer their children's questions about these subjects. Parents should keep careful watch on their children's behavior. Especially as they grow older, parents should be alert to any unusual mood changes, and encourage them to talk openly, heart-to-heart.

"You shall make a parapet"

"When you build a new house, you shall make a parapet for your roof, and you must not put blood upon your house, for someone might fall" (Deteronomy 22:8).

It is true that G-d watches over the details of people's lives and knows all their deeds and everything that is going to happen to them for good or bad according to His decree and His command in accordance with their merits or their guilt. As our Sages of blessed memory have said (*Chulin* 7a): "Nobody so much as knocks his finger in the lower world unless it is first announced in the upper world." At the same time, each person has a duty to protect himself against the chances of nature, for G-d created His world and built its foundations on the pillars of nature. He decreed that fire burns, while water puts out the blaze. Similarly, it inevitable by the laws of nature that if a large stone falls on someone's head, it will smash his brain, or if

---

a person falls from the top of a high roof to the ground, he will die. The Holy One, blessed be He, has given men the gift of their bodies and has breathed into each one's nostrils the soul of life, a soul gifted with the intelligence to protect the body from all harm. He has put the two of them - the soul and the body - under the wheel of nature and subjected them to its elements, which they are able to control and direct in order to accomplish what they need. Since G-d has put man's body under the rule of nature - for so His wisdom required, since man is a material being - He therefore commanded him to protect himself from natural dangers. For nature, into whose hands he has been given, will do what it is made to do against him if he will not protect himself from it.

Sefer HaChinuch Mitzvah #546

7 Food and Diet

"The Tzaddik eats to satisfy his soul" (Proverbs 13:25)

"Excessive intake of food is like poison to the human body and is the root cause of many illnesses. Most of the illnesses that strike people are caused either by bad foods or because people fill their stomachs with too much food, even when the foods are good. As King Solomon said in his wisdom: "One who guards his mouth and tongue keeps his soul from troubles" (Proverbs 21:23) - in other words, when he guards his mouth from eating bad foods or from overeating, and his tongue from speaking unnecessarily." (Rambam, Hilchos De'os 4:15)

"The main work of the doctors should be in the area of food and drink: to warn people what to avoid, and to give instructions about what to eat." (Ramban on Leviticus 26:11)

Good nutrition is one of the main foundations of physical and mental health. The body needs food to survive. Food is also the fuel of the mind and soul. Without food, the soul cannot remain in the body. The food we eat, and *how* we eat it, have a decisive influence on our health and the quality of our lives.

All our physical needs are provided by G-d, "in Whose hand is the soul of all living". Yet within the limitations of the *halachah*, G-d leaves us free to choose what we eat and how we eat it. The responsibility for our health and the quality of our lives is to a large extent in our own hands.

This a test! Adam's test was also in the realm of eating: he was forbidden to eat from the Tree of Knowledge. Because of his sin, he was condemned to eat by the sweat of his brow and eventually to die. Until today we have to make amends for Adam's failure. One of our tasks in life is to develop self-discipline in the way we eat: to choose healthy foods, and to eat them in the right way. This is our part in protecting our health and enhancing our life expectancy.

Taking care over what and how we eat is an inseparable part of the mitzvah of "Guard your souls", a mitzvah which is essentially about protecting ourselves from danger. Good nutrition not only prevents disease. It is also vital for healthy bodily and mental functioning and an overall feeling of wellbeing.

Poor nutrition is a danger to health. Prosperity has brought with it an abundance of food products that are rich in fats, sugars and artificial additives. The average daily diet is the cause of many health problems, especially obesity. Health experts attribute many cases of heart disease, cancer, diabetes, osteoporosis and other illnesses to poor diet. It can also cause many other physical and mental problems, including skin problems, allergic reactions, fatigue, tension, poor mental functioning, attention deficit, depression and behavioral problems.

In the wider world, the main emphasis in nutrition is on the components of the diet: what is healthy, what is unhealthy and what can cause harm. The outstanding Torah commentator Ramban (Nachmanides) bears this out in his comment that the main role of the doctor for Torah-observant Jews should be to give clear advice about what is healthy to eat and what is not.

More than this, it is impossible to provide a Jewish perspective on healthy nutrition without touching on the many mitzvos that are bound up with food. The Torah gives us detailed laws relating to all aspects of the growing and preparation of food, avoidance of forbidden foods, koshering meat, separating meat and milk, and so on. The Torah also gives us guidance about the actual eating of food, including washing the hands before bread, recital of blessings before and after eating, manners (*"Derech Eretz"*), Torah study and discussion during the meal. For the Jew, eating is an act of service and a way of coming closer to the Creator of the World. Eating and drinking are a central feature of Jewish life in the celebration of Shabbos (Kiddush, the three meals), on festivals (matzah on Pesach, eating in the Succah, feasting on Purim, etc. These mitzvos invest the eating of the Jew with sanctity and bring blessing into the food as it is digested and absorbed into his body.

"And you shall serve HaShem Your G-d, and He will bless your bread and your water, and I will remove illness from within you" (Exodus 23:25).

Know Him in all your ways

A person must have in mind that the ultimate goal of everything he does is only to know

---

G-d. The way he sits, stands, talks. everything should be directed to this purpose. How? When he eats and drinks his purpose should not be solely to enjoy himself, with the result that he eats only what is sweet to the palate. His intention should be to eat and drink for the sake of the health of his body and limbs. Therefore, he should not eat only what the palate craves, like a dog or a donkey. He should eat what is beneficial to the body, whether bitter or sweet, and he should not eat foods that are bad for the body, even when they are sweet to the palate. (Rambam, Hilchot De'ot 3:2)

Educating children in healthy nutrition

In the early years of life, healthy nutrition has a decisive influence on physical and mental growth and development, short-term and long term. All parents want the best for their children: so too in the area of nutrition. We try to feed our children in the best way possible. But feeding them well is not enough. As they grow, we must teach them good eating habits and explain the basic rules of healthy nutrition. With G-d's help, the education we give them will save them from many physical, mental and emotional problems and benefit them for many long years of good health and strength.

The best way to get the message across is by showing a good example. The food we eat at home and the way we eat it are the foundation of the children's education in good nutrition. We have an obligation to teach our children good eating habits just as we teach them to wash their hands before bread, to recite the blessings before and after food and to eat the Shabbos and Yom Tov meals.

We insist on kashrut of food without compromises. When we teach our children which foods are permitted and what is forbidden, we are also helping them develop self-discipline in eating. We must also teach them what foods are good for the body and what can cause harm. It is also desirable to give children a basic understanding of how the body's digestive system works to process the food, absorb the nutrients and expel the waste products. The purpose of this training is to prepare the children for the stage when they will have to make their own decisions about what and how to eat.

The urgency of nutritional education today

There has always been a natural human tendency to prefer foods that are tasty even when they are not the most healthy. The sophistication of contemporary food production and marketing makes the daily struggle with temptation harder than ever because of the abundance of appealing food products on the shelves of supermarkets, bakeries, snack and fast food stores, at simchahs and so on. Food manufacturers are primarily interested in persuading consumers to buy their products, which are often very attractive and appetite-whetting. But they are not always healthy, and some may even be harmful.

The battle against temptation is especially fierce when parents want to teach their children good nutrition. How is it possible to train children to eat a healthy diet when practically every day they are exposed to all kinds of candies and snack foods in *peklach* the receive when they go to Shul, on birthdays in the school or Cheder, at Siddur and Chumash parties, at simchahs and the like? What child is able to keep himself from eating the candies he has just been given when all his friends around him are already eating theirs? Can we ask the child at least to keep the candy until after his meal? Adults find it hard enough to resist temptation. How can children be expected to resist them, when the packaging, advertising, free gifts and "special offers" are directed straight at their soft hearts!

Are parents supposed to "have pity" on their children and allow them to eat all the sweets and candies they want, knowing they cause harm? Or should parents insist that their children eat only what is healthy, thereby putting them in an impossible position when all their friends are eating snacks and candies? How many times do parents give in after unremitting nagging by their children for something sweet? All too often the parents themselves are under pressure to find something to occupy the children or to stop them crying, and find a solution in giving them sweets and candies?!?

In practice, it is usually too much to expect that we can wean ourselves completely from unhealthy foods. Indeed, the truth is that as long as our daily diet is based on healthy, nutritious foods, it is not too bad if we occasionally eat less healthy foods for pleasure. As parents who want the best for our children, we must make every effort to provide them with a diet based on healthy foods, and we must teach them the importance of these foods. We must teach them that sweets, candies and similar snack-foods are not an alternative to healthy foods. They are a pleasant extra on special occasions, and even then, they should not be eaten to excess.

We, the parents, must be convinced of the importance of good nutrition, and we should learn and practice the basic principles. This is our main part in developing our children's awareness of good nutrition. Combined efforts by parents and teachers can make this work much easier.

It's not so hard

The rules of good nutrition are not as complicated or as limiting as they may seem. As soon as we start getting used to a new, improved diet, we will find that we have exchanged old pleasures for new ones, and our general feeling will undoubtedly improve. When we try to change eating habits, we are likely to encounter some difficulties. We should remember that what suits others may not necessarily be suitable for us. Each person must find the diet that suits his or her personally, and allow time to get used to it. We should not let ourselves become confused by the welter of conflicting nutritional advice we hear. The basic rules of good nutrition are very simple:

1. Eat a varied diet that includes foods from all the basic food categories rather than emphasizing only one kind of food. Each fruit and vegetable, every kind of grain and every other kind of food was created to make its unique contribution in providing nutrients needed by the body.

2. The main basis of the diet should be grains and grain-based foods, fruits, vegetables and legumes. Meat, fish, eggs and dairy products should make up a smaller proportion of the diet. As far as possible, consumption of fats and sugars should be limited. A properly balanced diet provides a steady supply of the main nutrients needed by the body.

3. Don't eat more than your body needs.

The main food groups

Different kinds of foods contain different combinations of nutrients and other beneficial substances. No single food can supply all the nutrients required by the body in the necessary amounts. Nutritionally, the different kinds of foods fall into six main groups. To provide the body with a good balance of nutrients and other healthful substances, choose a variety of foods from within and across the different food groups:

1. Bread, grains (e.g. rice, oats, breakfast cereals), pasta, etc.

2. Vegetables.

3. Fruits.

4. Milk, cheese, yogurt and other dairy products.

5. Meat, poultry, fish, beans, eggs and nuts.

6. Fats, oils and sweets.

Foods from the first group (bread and grains) together with those from the second and third (vegetables and fruits) make a sound basis for healthful diets. Choose a greater proportion of your foods from these groups. Eat more moderate quantities of foods in the milk and dairy group and of those in the meat, fish, eggs, beans and nuts group. Choose sparingly foods that are high in facts and sugars, for a diet that is excessively high in fats and sugars is a sure recipe for obesity, health problems and serious illnesses. Remember that many of the dishes you eat may contain foods from more than one group, such as soups or stews containing meat, beans, noodles and vegetables.

Bread and grains

Bread, grains (wheat, barley, oats, etc.) rice, pasta and other grain-based foods are a vital, positive source of energy for the body. All these foods contain carbohydrates, the "fuel" of the body. There are two types of carbohydrates: "complex" carbohydrates, as contained in the foods in this group, and "simple" carbohydrates, such as those in sugar. When the body receives simple carbohydrates in the form of candies, sweetened drinks and the like, the sugar is quickly absorbed into the blood, providing a fast, but temporary, boost of energy. The bodily immediately works to lower and balance the sugar levels in the blood, and as a result there is likely to be a quick, sharp drop in bodily energy, giving rise to cravings for more sugar to boost the energy again. And so the cycle continues. The advantage of foods from the group of grains and cereals is that they contain complex carbohydrates that are released into the body at a steady rate, keeping energy levels stable. This in itself gives a feeling of satisfaction, reducing overeating and food cravings between meals.

To increase the nutritional value of foods in the grains and cereals group, it is worth trying to use more grains in their natural form, such as whole wheat, whole oats, brown rice as well as baked products and pasta made of whole-grain flour. Grains in their husks are low in fats and rich in vitamins and dietary fiber, thereby helping reduce cholesterol and high blood sugar levels as well as aiding the movement of food through the digestive tract and the elimination of waste. (Note that grains must be carefully checked for worms and insects before use.)

Vegetables and fruits

Fresh vegetables and fruits are a most important component of the diet. They are especially rich in vitamins, minerals and other substances vital for healthy functioning and building of the body's immunity to illness. Vegetables and fruits provide complex carbohydrates and dietary fiber, giving energy and promoting healthy functioning of the digestive tract.

Fresh fruits and vegetables are a better choice than candies and snack foods when there is a need to eat between meals. Parents themselves will benefit from getting into the habit of eating fruits and vegetables when they want a snack, and they should teach their children to do the same.

Today pesticides are widely used in the cultivation of fruits and vegetables, which should be washed thoroughly before eating. Fruits and vegetables must also be checked carefully for worms and insects.

Milk and dairy products

Milk and dairy products (such as cheese, *leben,* yogurt, etc.) provide vital nutrients for the body, including protein and vitamins. They are especially important because of the rich supply of calcium they contain. Calcium is vital in the building of healthy bones, muscles and teeth, etc. and the prevention of osteoporosis. Everyone needs calcium, but it is especially important for babies, growing children and adolescents, all of whom need adequate supplies of calcium for healthy growth and development. Recent studies show that low bone density has become a widespread phenomenon among teenagers, and parents are advised to ensure that teenagers receive adequate calcium in their diet.

While the nutritional value of milk products is high, their proportion in the overall diet should be lower than that of foods in the grains, vegetables and fruits groups. Excess consumption of dairy products that are high in fat should be avoided. Dairy products that are high in added sugar should be reserved for special occasions.

Meat, poultry, fish, eggs, legumes, nuts and seeds

The main importance of meat, poultry, fish, eggs, legumes, nuts and seeds in the diet lies in the fact that they provide protein, essential in building the cells of the body and vital to overall healthy functioning. The proportion of foods from this group in a healthy diet should be less than that of grains, vegetables and fruits. But remember that an adequate supply of proteins is especially important for babies, children and adolescents. When the diet includes meat or poultry, it is preferable to use those parts of the animal or bird that are lower in fat. Likewise, eggs should not be eaten to excess as they have a high cholesterol content.

Worms and insects are frequently found in nuts, seeds, beans and the like, and they should be carefully checked before use.

Fats and Sugars

The body needs fats and sugar - in the right amounts. Most basic foods -- grains, fruits and vegetables, meat, fish and dairy -- contain fats, sugars or both in various forms. Meat contains fat, milk contains fat and sugar, fruits, vegetable and grains contain sugars. A good, basic daily diet can provide all the sugar and fats the body requires without any need for the added sugar and fats contained in many man-made foods.

Yet it is human nature to love rich, sweet foods. Throughout history, people have sought ways of satisfying this desire over and above what the body needs. Satisfaction of this desire is one of the main foundations of much of the food industry, which in our technological age has grown to gigantic proportions, using the most sophisticated methods of food production and marketing to appeal to consumers' palates. How healthy are all these food products?

Many of the foods and drinks filling the shelves of supermarkets, bakeries, snack and fast food stores, etc., contain high quantities of added fats and sugars. Sometimes this may be fairly obvious, but in other cases the added fat and sugar content may not be apparent to the average consumer. Much of the food we prepare at home -- fried foods, cakes and biscuits, desserts, etc. -- are not exactly low in fats and sugars!

The problem begins when the extra fats and sugars become a regular component of the daily diet. When the body receives more of these nutrients than it can use, bodily balance is upset. This can express itself in different ways. Excess fat intake leads to all the problems of becoming overweight and high cholesterol in the blood, which thickens artery walls and causes heart disease. Cycles of excessive sugar intake followed by cravings for more sugar may lead to diabetes as well as causing other problems. Excess fat and sugar in the diet can interfere with the body's ability to absorb important vitamins and minerals (including calcium) even when the diet is rich in these nutrients. This is a particular problem in the case of children and teenagers in various stages of development.

The obvious conclusion is that excess consumption of fats and sugars is the leading cause of some of the most serious health problems and illnesses in our time, such as heart and arterial disease, diabetes, cancer, osteoporosis and other degenerative diseases. In order to protect ourselves and avoid these problems with G-d's help, we should make every effort to base our daily diet on foods in the grain, vegetable and fruits groups while limiting consumption of foods with a high fat and sugar content.

We must understand -- and we must teach our children -- that there is a difference between the foods we eat to keep healthy, which must be the basis of our daily diet, as opposed to the foods we eat mainly for pleasure, which should be reserved for special occasions.

"And you shall call Shabbos a delight" (Isaiah 58:13). It is a mitzvah to honor Shabbos and festivals with special foods and drinks -- "to delight with pleasures...with all kinds of tasty foods... fragrant wines, dainty treats." (from the Shabbos *Zemiros*) -- in order to delight the body and soul. It is a good idea to reserve eating the richer, sweeter foods for Shabbos, festivals, celebrations and other special occasions. And even then, we shouldn't overdo it!

Salt

Salt is needed by the body in limited quantities in order to maintain fluid balance and stabilize blood pressure. Salt improves and enhances the taste of food, but for this very reason it is easy to cross the red line in salt consumption. Many artificial and processed foods have a high salt (or sodium) content. Health experts consider the salt content of the average diet to be considerably higher than necessary. Excessive consumption of salt can cause high blood pressure.

Vitamins and food supplements

Vitamins, minerals and other food supplements may have a role to play in certain cases of nutritional deficiency. However, man-made supplements cannot provide the basic daily nutrients our bodies need in the same balanced way as our food. Normally, people who eat a healthy diet that includes a variety of foods from the main food groups in the proper quantities should not need to take food supplements on a regular basis. A doctor or nutritionist can advise when supplements are needed.

What to drink

Water has a role in all our main bodily processes. Water is the main component of our blood and all our other bodily fluids. Water plays a vital role in digesting our food and bringing nutrients to all the cells in our bodies. Likewise, water places a crucial role in the removal of waste products from the body, in overall metabolism, regulates the heat of the body and other important functions. The body cannot survive without water!

Our bodies lose water constantly through breathing, in the form of sweat, in the urine and stools, etc. To maintain the balance of fluids in the body, it is necessary to replace this lost water by drinking. Many of the foods we eat, especially fruits and vegetables, contain water, but the quantities are normally insufficient to supply all the body's needs. This is why it is important to drink as well.

The healthiest drink of all is water itself. Milk and fruit juices are healthful, but should not be relied upon as the main source of fluid intake. Sweetened drinks, colas and the like must not be allowed to take the place of water in supplying fluids.

Excessive consumption of such drinks is harmful. Excess consumption of coffee and other caffeine-containing beverages is also harmful.

As parents we have an obligation to teach our children not to ignore feelings of thirst and to drink enough to meet the needs of the body. This applies particularly after intense physical activity and in hot weather. Children should be taught about the dangers of fluid deficiency and dehydration, and that these can be avoided by drinking sufficiently, avoiding extended periods of exposure to the sun and wearing proper clothing.

Good eating habits

"A person's table is his altar of atonement" (*Berachos* 55a)

At the center of the Jewish home, a miniature sanctuary, stands the table, which our sages compared to the Temple altar. In the Temple, items from the animal, vegetable and inanimate world became sacrifices, "A fire offering, a pleasing savor to HaShem" (Leviticus 1:9). In our very homes we have the power to elevate the food we eat to the level of a sacrificial offering when we sanctify the strength it gives us to the service of G-d, study of His Torah, prayer and performance of the mitzvos. This applies every day and especially when we eat on Shabbos and festivals. Washing our hands, saying the blessings before and after the food and conducting ourselves in the proper manner during meals turn the physical eating of the Jew into an act of holy service.

"At first the Children of Israel were like chickens pecking in the garbage, until Moses came and gave them fixed mealtimes" (*Yoma* 75a). This and other sayings of our Sages underline the importance of eating regular meals. Regular meals correctly spaced through the day and based on the main food groups in the proper proportions supply the body with the proper nutrients at the proper times for optimal, healthy functioning. Regular, balanced meals, give a feeling of satisfaction that reduces the need to eat between meals. The rabbis placed particular emphasis on *Pas Shacharis*, a morning breakfast of bread or grains. This provides a steady supply of energy and contributes to sound bodily and mental functioning.

When planning children's diet, it is essential to remember that they are growing and developing, and their nutritional needs are different from those of adults. Children's stomachs are smaller and more delicate, and they need smaller meals at more frequent intervals. For the same reason they should not be prevented from eating between meals. When children need to eat between meals, it is preferable to give them fruits, vegetables, nuts and seeds etc. rather than candies and the like.

As they grow older, children should be taught to eat the foods that provide the main nutrients they need during their regular meals. Parents should make every effort to provide nutritious, tasty meals so as to reduce the need for "extras", especially candies, between meals.

The parental responsibility to keep watch over what their children are eating does not end when they enter puberty and advance into their teen years. Quite often it is precisely at this age that problems of excess weight begin to develop, and these may present serious health threats later on. Such problems are increasingly widespread among students who study for long hours with limited opportunities for physical activity. Parents of children with an inclination to excess weight should seek ways of helping them find the proper balance between adequate nutrition and physical activity.

At the table

1. Just as we insist that our children wash their hands properly before they eat and say the blessings correctly, we should also insist on good habits when they eat. Good table habits increase the body's ability to digest and absorb the food properly.

2. Eat sitting down.

3. Do not put too much food into the mouth at once.

4. Chew the food well.

5. Stop eating before you feel too full.

6. It is best not to drink too much with the meal. Wait until the food starts being digested (about 20 minutes) and then drink as much as you need, though not too much.

7. Don't engage in demanding physical activity directly after a meal: wait until the food is digested.

Education in *Derech Eretz* and good table manners should be an inseparable part of children's education in proper eating habits. For a Jew the purpose of eating is not merely to keep the body alive. The essential purpose is to serve G-d. It is not enough to eat healthy foods. We must be aware that our food is provided by G-d, "Who sustains the whole world with grace, kindness and mercy." We must behave appropriately when we eat at the table of the King! The mitzvos we perform, the blessings we recite and our manners and behavior when we eat, together with the healthy food, turn the physical function of eating into an act of holy service. In the merit of this service, we will turn our table into an altar and see in our own lives fulfillment of G-d's promise that "He will bless your bread and your water, and remove illness from among you".

Fixed mealtimes

The Rabbis taught: ...The fourth hour of the day is the time for most people to eat their morning meal. The fifth hour is mealtime for workers. The sixth hour is mealtime for Torah scholars. Eating the first meal of the

---

day from that time on is like throwing a stone into an empty bottle. (*Shabbos* 11a).

When the fourth hour arrives, one should sit down to his meal. A Torah scholar who is busy studying may wait till the sixth hour. One should not eat the meal any later, as it's like throwing a stone into an empty bottle if one has eaten nothing all morning. (*Shulchan Aruch, Orach Chaim* #157)

In praise of morning bread (*Pas Shacharis*)

...Eighty-three illnesses are caused by gall bladder problems, and Morning Bread (*Pas Shacharis*) with salt and a flagon of water prevents them all. The rabbis taught: Thirteen things were said of morning bread. It saves a person from the sun, from chills, draughts and bad spirits, it gives wisdom to the simple, the person wins his case, it helps the person learn and teach Torah, his words are heard, he remembers what he has learned, his body does not give odors, he loves his wife and has no desire for any other women. Morning bread kills parasites in the intestines and some say it removes jealousy and makes the person feel love. (*Bava Metzia* 107a).

Halachos of Eating

A person should not eat and drink greedily. One should not eat standing or drink standing. The table should be clean and covered nicely even if one does not intend to eat a full meal. One should not hold too large a piece of food in one's hand and eat from it. Nor should one hold the food in one hand and pull off pieces to eat with the other hand.

One should not take a bite from a piece of food and put the rest back on the table, give it to someone else or put it on his plate, because this may be off-putting to the other person. Nor should one drink from a cup and give the rest to someone else to drink.

Do not talk while eating - even words of Torah - as it could be dangerous if the food goes into the windpipe instead of the gullet. However, when not actually eating, it a mitzvah to say words of Torah at the table, and one should be very careful to do so.

It is forbidden to throw bread, even where it will not be spoiled, because throwing bread is disrespectful. Other foods that could be spoiled should also not be thrown.

Kitzur Shulchan Aruch #42

8 Physical Activity and Exercise

"As long as a person exercises and exerts himself a lot, takes care not to eat to the point of being completely full, and keeps his bowels soft, illness will not come upon him and his strength will increase. And whoever sits comfortably and takes no exercise. even if he eats the best foods and follows healthcare principles in other areas of his life, all his days will be full of pain and his strength will decline."

Maimonides, Hilchot Deot 4:15

Daily physical activity together with sound nutrition is the best formula for a healthy lifestyle.

The greatest doctors, headed by the outstanding giant in Torah and healing, the RaMBaM (Rabbi Moshe ben Maimon, Maimonides (1135-1204), have always recommended regular physical activity involving effort as being vital to health. Such activity promotes the development of strong bones, strong, flexible muscles and joints that allow free, easy, unrestricted movement. Regular sustained physical activity makes the the functioning of the body's respiratory and blood circulation systems more efficient, providing stable supplies of oxygen and nutrients to all parts of the body and enhancing overall metabolism. Physical activity also aids the digestive system and the elimination of waste products from the body.

Improved functioning gives the body greater powers of endurance in everyday activities while storing energy for emergencies. When a person is fit, the person *feels* better, physically and mentally, and can stand up better under pressure.

Similarly, the dangers of many illnesses are considerably reduced - "Illness will not come upon him, and his strength will increase."

Lack of regular physical activity causes the muscles to become weak and flabby. The joints become stiff and more injury-prone, and the lungs, heart and blood circulation become less efficient. The problems become more serious when we eat more than the body needs, and then the excess food turns into deposits of fat in various parts of the body. Excess fat caused by imbalance between intake of foods and physical activity is the leading cause of heart and other serious diseases today.

The importance of exercise today

In the past, before the development of modern technology, most people's daily routine involved considerable physical activity, including walking and various kinds of labor involving bodily movement and effort. It might seem that they should not have needed additional physical exercise for the sake of their health. Yet Rambam, writing over eight hundred years ago, stated definitively: "As long as a person exercises and exerts himself a lot, illness will not come upon him and his strength will increase." Even then, Rambam saw the need to emphasize the importance of physical activity to health - which means it's even more important today!

Means of transport, sophisticated machines and electrical equipment that does our work for us at the push of a button have made our lives easier in amazing ways. But by saving us a considerable amount of physical effort, they have taken from us many natural opportunities to use and exercise our bodies. The problem is especially great among those whose daily "activity" is mostly sitting, including office workers, drivers and students in Yeshiva. Added to the problem is today's average daily diet, which is richer than in the past, especially in fats and sugars. Inadequate physical activity and unhealthy diet are at the root of many of the health problems and illnesses with which people today are afflicted.

Today, it is more important than ever to set regular times in our daily schedule for some kind of health-promoting physical activity. The need is even greater for those of us whose day involves limited physical activity. Each one of us needs to find the right kind of activities that will help us to maintain and enhance our bodily fitness and reduce the risks of illness.

In the wider world there is ever-growing awareness of the need for extra physical activity and a heavy investment in activities whose declared purpose is improving fitness, health-maintenance and prevention of illness. Yet in fact, the pursuit of these goals has turned into a culture of its own that puts the main emphasis on cultivation of the body and bodily appearance and its ability to derive the greatest enjoyment from life. This culture has spawned a complete industry of sports events, media coverage, advertising, fitness centers, equipment, factories, stores and so on, involving enormous sums of money.

Sport and exercise become idolatry when their essential goal is development of the body and physical fitness for the sole sake of enjoying the material pleasures of life. For Jews who keep the Torah and the Mitzvos, the true purpose of engaging in the physical activities that promote health is to make the body a fit instrument for the service of G-d.

> If only a person would care for himself the way he cares for the animal he rides on, he would be saved from many bad illnesses. You will not find anyone who gives his animal more food than necessary. He measures out the animal's feed according to what the animal can take, but he himself eats to excess without measure and without a thought. Similarly, he calculates how much exercise and activity his animal needs to keep fit and not become sick. But the person himself does not apply this to his own body, and gives little thought to exercise, even though it is the key to maintaining health and avoiding most illnesses, and there is no other substitute whatever for physical activity and exercise.
>
> *Rambam*, Guide to Health 1,3

What is exercise?

Many people think that keeping fit requires hard exercises and sophisticated equipment. This is a mistake! Many simple activities can be equally if not more effective in promoting health than many popular kinds of exercise. For example, a brisk 20-30 minute walk three or four times a week can provide the quota of physical activity necessary to maintain fitness better than a complicated exercise system.

The Rambam in his well-known *Hanhagas HaBri'us*, "The Guide to Health" (1,3), defines the kind of physical activity that is healthy in the following way: "Exercise is a form of activity involving bodily movements that may be strong or gentle or a combination of the two and which cause changes in the person's breathing, which becomes more rapid." The Rambam's definition corresponds to the "aerobic" exercise recommended by present-day specialists, a steady, non-stop activity that involves a certain degree of effort and leads to increased rates of blood circulation and breathing without putting strain on the heart and lungs. Brisk walking is one such activity, stimulating the blood circulation without putting a strain on the breathing. Other examples include running (even in place), dancing, swimming, etc. To achieve the desired results, the activity should be sustained for up to 40 minutes and no less than 15 minutes, and it should be carried out 3-4 times a week. Activity of this kind increases the body's ability to keep up physical activity and effort for sustained periods.

Other kinds of physical movements that have an important role in keeping us fit and healthy are those that require various body parts to apply force against some kind of resistance, exercising the muscles and increasing their strength and endurance. While weight-lifting and exercise machines may be used for this kind of exercise, many everyday activities provide opportunities for the kind of movements that are beneficial to health, such as climbing stairs rather than using an elevator, carrying shopping, many kinds of house work and even kneading dough.

Movements that involve stretching different parts of the body are also important in developing muscle and joint flexibility, giving increased freedom of movement and contributing to a relaxed bodily feeling. Such movements also reduce the danger of muscle and joint injuries, including pulled muscles and sprains.

Each person needs to find the kinds of exercises that are suit him or her personally. Exercise can help in many cases of neck, shoulder and back pain as well as other physical problems. It is worth raising the subject with your doctor.

Physical activity for children

G-d gives most people the gift of physical fitness and flexibility in their childhood, but this precious gift is easily lost unless we ourselves take proper care of it. The best way to protect our health is by developing healthy habits from the earliest age, of which one of the most vital is regular exercise.

The need for physical activity begins in childhood. Physical activity is essential to build strong bones and muscles, maintain muscle and joint flexibility and develop the endurance of the respiratory and blood circulation systems. The positive effects of healthy levels of physical activity in children are seen immediately, while the long-term benefits include general strength and flexibility, healthy blood pressure, healthy weight, overall good feeling, confidence and a willingness to get the best out of what God has granted us, physically and mentally.

People often imagine children as being active and busy running, climbing, jumping and playing - but in fact, the picture is not accurate. Many children are not sufficiently physically active. Children who do not have sufficient opportunities to exercise their bodies become tired, lazy and indifferent. It is our duty to teach our children the importance of physical activity and to provide them with suitable opportunities.

The need for physical activity by children on a regular basis starts at the age of about two. The activity should be in the form of "play". One of the best places for healthy play is on the play equipment in the public park. There is no need for the child to feel he is involved in "physical activity": he plays and enjoys himself. The most beneficial games are those that require greater physical effort than regular activities, such as those that involve running, jumping, climbing and so on. When it is not possible to play on play equipment, parents should use their imaginations in providing the children with healthy activities. For good results, the activity should continue for at least 15-30 minutes, several times a week. Children's play should be under supervision to avoid accidents.

Older children and teenagers

The need for physical activity continues and indeed increases as children grow older and enter puberty and adolescence. The need of girls for physical activity may be met with games like skipping rope and other children's games, movement and dance. Household tasks involving some kind of physical effort - from washing floors to kneading dough - also fulfil part of the need for physical exercise.

In the case of boys and young men who spend much of their day sitting studying Torah, the need for additional physical activity is greater. Not only will this contribute to their health and fitness, it will also increase their alertness, concentration and ability to think. As the boys grow older, their hours of study are longer, and their free time becomes increasingly limited. Parents must help them to take advantage of simple, everyday activities to give their bodies exercise.

Encourage your children to go on foot instead of by bus etc. when this is possible, to climb the stairs instead of using the elevator, and so on.

Help your children make it a habit to take a brisk walk for at least 15-20 minutes 3-4 times a week. Friends can go in pairs or groups at a pace that is sufficiently relaxed to allow for conversation without being too slow. Students can use the time spent walking mentally reviewing their studies, listening to a class on a walkman or thinking their thoughts.

Consult with a doctor or fitness specialist about simple exercises for strength, flexibility and general fitness.

Use vacation times (*Bein Haz'manim*) for physical activities that time does not permit during the rest of the year. It would be desirable if more educational institutions would organize camps of the kind that combine swimming and holiday activities with study in a relaxed environment.

Encourage the children to dance energetically on Simchas Torah and other joyous celebrations. Dancing is good for the body and the soul!

Breathing

Regular deep breathing helps supply the body with flesh oxygen and stimulates blood circulation. This refreshes and energizes the body, making us more alert and energetic, and at the same time more relaxed. Many people's breathing is too shallow, leading to a loss of energy and clarity, nervousness and lowered resistance to illness.

Parents should learn the following simple breathing exercise and teach it to their children: breathe in steadily, letting the lungs swell with air until they are full to capacity. Hold the air in the lungs for a few seconds, then release it in a slow, complete exhalation. Ten slow, deep breaths before going to sleep, on rising in the morning, when feeling tired, at times of strain or on any other occasion provide immediate relaxation and stimulation.

The Benefits of Exercise

1. Physical activity "burns" calories. When we burn more calories than we take in, we automatically reduce weight.

2. Activities involving physical effort (even climbing the stairs instead of using the elevator) strengthen muscles and bones and increase the body's endurance during periods of sustained activity.

3. Movements involving stretching of various body parts promote muscle and joint flexibility, and help the body feel relaxed. They also reduce the risks of muscle and joint injuries (e.g. pulled muscles, sprains).

4. Sustained physical activity (between 15-30 minutes) such as brisk walking, running in place and dance, improve the functioning of the lungs and heart, stimulate the blood circulation and increase the body's endurance during periods of sustained activity.

5. Physical exercise enhances overall bodily functioning and strengthens immunity against illness.

6. Regular fitness activities improve the quality of life, bring increased strength and stamina, reduce tension and anxiety, promote healthy sleep and relax the body and the mind.

9 Sleep, Rest and Relaxation

"If a person sleeps in order to allow his mind to rest and to give rest to his body so that he should not become sick and unable to serve G-d because of illness, in this case his very sleep is service of G-d. This is the meaning of the precept of the sages that 'all your deeds should be for the sake of heaven'" (Rambam, Hilchos Deos 3, 3).

Good sleep is as important as good nutrition!

Almost a third of our lives are spent asleep! Sleep is vital to bodily functioning. When a person has enough healthy sleep, he is fresh, his mind functions better, his moods are better and his ability to achieve his goals, material and spiritual, is greatly enhanced. Developing healthy habits of sleep is also a part of the mitzvah of "Take care of your souls" -- "...his very sleep is service of G-d!"

In the opinion of the Rambam and the Ben Ish Chai (1835-1909), the average adult needs between six to eight hours of sleep a night. Regularly sleeping for more than eight hours a night can be no less harmful than regularly getting less than six hours sleep a night. The results of extensive research conducted recently in sleep laboratories bear out the recommendations of these great Torah sages.

In the case of children, the need for sleep is greater. Children need sleep not only to rest from today and gain strength for tomorrow; sleep is vital to their proper growth and development. Most of a baby's time is spent sleeping. As the baby grows, he sleeps less. Medical experts recommend that children between the ages of 5 and 12 should have an average of 8-10 hours of sleep a night. The need for sleep continues to become less, until it balances out at 6-8 hours a night.

Children and sleep

We all know that many adults would be only too happy to have more hours of sleep, but it can be very hard to persuade children to go to sleep! Too often the children finally drop, totally exhausted, late at night -- and the resulting fatigue is felt very well the next day. The child is so tired that he falls asleep during the day, goes to bed late again that night, gets up tired the next morning. and so the vicious cycle continues. All kinds of occasions and other factors contribute to the problem: simchah celebrations, special events, the summertime clock and more.

The difference between sufficient, healthy night-time sleep and short, interrupted night-time sleep makes itself felt in the child's behavior the next day. After a good night's sleep, the child gets up in the morning rested, refreshed, full of energy, smiling, nicely-behaved, able to think and concentrate. But when a child doesn't sleep enough at night, he gets up tired and is likely to be nagging, irritable, drowsy unable to think and concentrate and badly-behaved. School studies suffer, and this is a loss that cannot easily be made up.

We all know that preparing children for bed at night is a continual battle where we have to try to persuade them not only to get into bed but also to fall asleep. The key to success is routine. Parents should do everything in their power to organize themselves in such a way that they have fixed times to feed the children their evening meal, prepare them for going to sleep and get them into bed. It helps when the parents spend a little time with the children when they are already in bed, whether to talk to them or tell them a relaxing story. This helps prepare the children mentally to go to sleep. There is plenty of scope for us to use our imagination here!

Adolescents and teenagers

The struggle to make sure our children get enough sleep takes a new form as they enter puberty and advance into their teens. Their studies take up long hours and the time remaining for other activities is limited. The result is that sleep is often pushed low down on their order of priorities. It's not so bad if they don't get enough sleep once in a while, but if it becomes a habit, the effects can be serious: tiredness, poor concentration, impaired thinking, weak memory, lack of alertness in class, poor mood and irritability as well as the negative effects on physical development.

Adolescents and teenagers are naturally more independent. Indeed, it is important to encourage them to be independent -- as long as we also teach them to act responsibly. At the same time, parents need to continue keeping watch over their children without trying to control them and without hurting their feelings. With regard to sleep, if teenagers diverge too far from healthy patterns, parents should gently help them establish a better routine.

Some ways to encourage healthy sleep

1. Have a regular bedtime routine and try to arrange your schedule so you can keep to it.

2. Simchah-celebrations, special events, an unexpected visit to the doctor and much else may come up force changes from the regular schedule, delaying bedtime. Instead of sleeping too late next morning, it causes less of a disruption to the regular routine if one gets up as near as possible to the usual time and then goes to bed earlier that evening. This applies to both adults and children.

3. During the day, it can be highly refreshing to close the eyes and take half an hour of deep bodily relaxation without going to sleep. It is best not to sleep for long during the day as this interferes with the next night's sleep, and the effects will be felt the following day.

4. After a meal it is best to wait until the food is digested before going to sleep -- when the body is busy digesting the food, the sleep is not healthy.

5. From the late afternoon onwards, it is advisable to avoid coffee, colas and other drinks that contain caffeine, which keeps most people awake.

6. Physical activity and exercise during the day are stimulating and invigorating, and also contribute to relaxed sleep at night. It is unadvisable to engage in intense physical activity immediately before going to bed.

7. Leave time to unwind before going to sleep. Keep the lights low - bright light is good in the morning, but avoid it in the evening as it signals the brain that it's time to wake up.

People sometimes find they become very drowsy at certain points during the day and it becomes an effort to keep their eyes open even when they have had enough sleep. This can often be a problem with young students. In some cases, such problems may be related to what they are eating, when and how. For example, a rich evening meal before going to sleep followed by a large breakfast in the morning can give rise to feelings of heaviness and drowsiness. There are some foods that make certain people sleepy. This is an individual matter. Simple changes in eating habits may help correct the problem.

The day and night are twenty-four hours. It is sufficient for a person to sleep one third of that time, namely eight hours. This should be in the latter part of the night so that from the time one goes to sleep until the sun comes up is eight hours. This way one rises from one's bed before the sun comes up. One should not sleep flat on one's face nor flat on one's back but rather on one's side, at the beginning of the night on the left side and at the end of the night on the right side. One should not go to sleep directly after eating but wait from three to four hours, and one should not sleep by day. (Rambam, Hilchos Deos 4, 4-5).

How much sleep?

One should not think that the more a person sleeps, the better it is for the body. All leading doctors agree that a person should sleep at night no less than six hours and no more than eight, because too much sleep is harmful. All the doctors agree that sleeping for more than eight hours is harmful to the body, whereas a person who sleeps for six hours completely fulfills the duty he has to take proper care of the health of his body. For this reason, a Jew -- who is also obliged to take proper care of the health of his holy soul -- should sleep no more than six hours. This way, he fulfills his obligation to protect the health of his body, and he should spend the remaining hours of the night engaged in Torah in order to promote the health of his soul. And if, on occasion, he sleeps less than the six hours that are for the health of his body, adding to the hours he spends cultivating the health of his soul, he can be sure that his physical health will not suffer in any way. For this reason, on Thursday nights, the night before the New Moon, during the month of Elul, the Ten Days of Penitence and so on, if a person sleeps for less than six hours, he can be sure that his bodily health will not suffer any way.

When is the best time to sleep?

Although the whole night is a time for sleep, nevertheless, it is better to sleep during the first half of the night and not during the second. This has benefits on both the physical plane -- it is healthier for the body -- and also on the spiritual plane -- it helps in the rectification of the soul and all the worlds. A leading doctor has written: "From midnight to midday is like a person's age of ascent; from midday until the evening is like his time of stability, while the time from the evening until midnight may be compared to his days of decline. Therefore, a person who stays awake during the first half of the night and sleeps during the second half of the night is like someone who is active during the days of decline while resting during the age of ascent. In the holy work, *Ru'ach Chaim* "Spirit of Life" (p. 90), a famous sage is quoted as having said: "Going to bed in the early evening and rising in the early morning make a person healthy, wise and strong." It is also good for women who always have several hours of work to do at night to get into the habit of sleeping in the first part of the night and rising very early to do their work: "And she rises while it is yet night and gives prey to her house" (Proverbs 31:15).

Ben Ish Chai I, *Vayishlach* 1

Resting the eyes

Sometimes, we feel tired not so much because our bodies are tired as because our *eyes* are tired. The eyes are the most delicate, active parts of our bodies. We use them all day and a good part of the night in natural and artificial light. Students, those who work in front of computer screens and many others, often need to use their eyes intensively for many hours. If we strain our eyes for prolonged periods without resting them, it is hardly surprising if the strain and tiredness makes our vision blurred. People often think this must be because of bad eyesight, and run to test their vision.

In many cases of poor vision there is little choice but to use suitable glasses. It is important to have not only a vision test but also a thorough eye examination by a specialist. However, many people experience difficulties in seeing not so much because of any fault in the physical structure of their eyes but because of the way they *use* their eyes. If we consider how the eye works, we will see that some visual problems can be avoided easily with simple techniques.

The eye is a receiver of light. For that reason, the best way to see is when the light is good -- it is particularly important to read in good light, not in semi-darkness or when the page is in shadow. When it comes to resting and relaxing the eyes, we do it by shutting out the light. The main way we rest our eyes is when we close them to sleep at night in the dark. Yet even with a proper quota of sleep, our eyes need periods of rest from use throughout the day. Today the need for this is greater than ever before: artificial lighting has increased our eyes' "working hours", while the "workload" is greater because of the flood of reading material.

Our eyelids were created to protect our eyes and also to give them rest, even momentarily, every time we blink. Often when concentrating intently on reading, there is a tendency to stare at the words and blink less. This deprives the eyes of their natural rest. It's good to blink!

When reading for lengthy periods it is advisable to lift the eyes from the page from time to time and look at a far-off object. This gives the eye relief from the tension caused by prolonged focussing on the text. From time to time it is good to practice switching focus from near objects to far and from far to near -- this helps maintain the eyes' focussing ability.

Palming

One of the simplest and most effective ways of relaxing the eyes is by covering them for a short time with the palms of the hands. This can be especially helpful at points in the day when our eyes feel tired and strained -- it can help us prepare to get back to work again refreshed, with clearer vision and renewed powers of concentration.

Rest your elbows on a desk or table, close your eyes and cover them with your hands so that your palms are covering your eyes while your fingers are extended over your forehead up to the scalp. While leaning gently on your arms, rest your eyes lightly against your palms, cupping them a little to avoid pressing on the eyes. The idea is to shut out as much light as possible to rest the eyes. The warmth of the palms of the hands relaxes the eyes and surrounding muscles.

Palming may be practiced as needed for periods of anywhere from 1-2 minutes to 10-15 minutes or even longer if your eyes are particularly strained. It can be done anywhere and at any time. Particularly when you have a lot of work to do but feel eye-strain and fatigue, covering your eyes for a few minutes can be very refreshing. Practiced at the end of the day before going to bed it can make your sleep more restful and refreshing.

This simple exercise is so beneficial that it is well worth teaching it to children at a young age. It can help them relax their eyes and may assist in avoiding short- and long-term vision problems. Palming is particularly helpful at the age when children spend more of their time reading and writing, which is when children often complain of having difficulty seeing.

The exercise can be practiced in the classroom and at home, singly and in a group. In addition to its beneficial effects on vision, sitting quietly for a while helps children relax. When practiced in a group, it can be a time for being "together", telling a story, talking about something interesting or playing question and answer games. Older students can put the time spent resting their eyes to good use to mentally review their studies, examine and work on themselves, offer some personal prayers, listen to a tape or just relax.

Care of the ears

Sh'ma Yisrael! Hear, Israel! We depend on our ears when saying and listening to our words of prayer, studying the Torah, hearing what's going on around us and communicating with one another to transmit and receive information, thoughts and feelings. Our ears are also extremely delicate. For all these reasons, it is important to take proper care of our ears, and as parents, we must communicate this to our children.

Never insert *anything* (finger, pen or even cotton swabs) in the ears, for this can easily hurt the ear, make it bleed or even cause an ear infection. When washing children's heads, try to avoid getting water in their ears, and if water does get in, dry them carefully with a towel.

Protect the ears from excessive noise, including very loud music from speakers or headphones. Exposure to noise can harm our hearing. When we know we are likely to be exposed to loud noise, it is a good idea to use protective earplugs.

In cases of persistent ear pain or any other ear problem, even the slightest, consult a doctor.

May we guard our ears, physically and spiritually, and merit fulfillment of the promise in the Torah:

"**If you will surely** *hear* **the voice of HaShem your G-d. and listen to His commandments.** *all the diseases that I have put upon the Egyptians, I will not put upon you, for I, HaShem am your Healer*" **(Exodus 15:26).**

10 The Joy of Living

"Serve G-d with joy." (Psalms 100:2)

"And I praised joy" (Kohelet 8:15) - this is the joy of a mitzvah. "And what does joy accomplish?" (ibid. 2:2) - this refers to happiness which is not bound up with a mitzvah, to teach you that the Divine Presence dwells not out of sadness, laziness, frivolity, light-headedness, chatter and idle pursuits but through the joy of a mitzvah, as it is written: "'And now, bring me a musician', and when the musician played, the spirit of G-d rested upon him" (II Kings, 3:15). (*Shabbos 30a*)

"It is a mitzvah to bring the Divine Presence to rest upon us" (Rashi ad loc.)

The body cannot survive without the soul. Taking proper care of the body is only one side of a healthy lifestyle. Equally, if not more important is to take proper care of the mind and soul! The best indicator of mental and emotional health is *Simchah* -- a happy, positive approach to life. This is what gives us the incentive to make the best of life!

Many of us are well aware of the basic rules of healthy living: which foods are good and which are harmful, how important it is to exercise, how dangerous it is to smoke. Even so, we keep on finding ourselves doing exactly the opposite! We eat too much of the wrong foods. We prefer to take things easy instead of exerting ourselves. We ride instead of walking. We smoke. Why???

In many cases, the things that impel us are psychological: pressures in the home and outside, tension, anxiety, insecurity, boredom, anger, and so on. When we continue eating even after we are full, or snack between meals, it is often because of inner tension, depression, anger or boredom. The same factors often make people act carelessly and put themselves in danger. Depression and despair can make people neglect their bodies and loose interest in taking proper care of their health.

If we really want to take care of our bodies and cultivate a healthy lifestyle, first and foremost we must get to the roots of the inner mental and emotional factors that drive us in the opposite direction.

Today there is an abundance of techniques intended to help people deal with problems like stress, anxiety and depression through relaxation, medications, herbal remedies, biofeedback, homeopathy and many others. While these techniques may help, the best foundation of all is an ancient technique that has proved itself throughout history: Faith! When a person has faith, he has a wellspring of inner power that will strengthen his resolve to go and make the effort needed to improve his life.

Who knows this better than the Jews, and especially those who keep the Torah and mitzvos! When we know and believe that the Creator of the World is watching over us at every moment and that He is the one who provides us with all our needs, we know that there is no reason to worry. We have to do our part, but we do not have to be frantic! Our main efforts should be directed at keeping the Torah and the mitzvos -- including the mitzvah of "Guard yourself" -- as our sages have taught us. When we do what is incumbent upon us, we can rest assured that G-d will not stop watching over us for a single moment - "And he who trusts in G-d, kindness will surround him" (Psalms 32:10).

As parents seeking to help our children follow a healthy lifestyle, we must keep in mind that developing a positive attitude based on faith and trust in G-d is the best foundation for cultivating healthy habits. What our children learn in their early years will determine their future approach to the mitzvah of safeguarding their health physically, mentally and spiritually: "Educate the youth according to his way, even when he grows old, he will not turn from it" (Proverbs 22:6). We must inculcate our children with the faith and trust that G-d never ceases to watch over us, and He promises us:

"If you will serve HaShem your G-d, He will bless your bread and your water, and I will remove illness from within you." Amen.

Tips for developing a positive attitude

Looking for the good: No matter what you may be up against, try to look on the good side of things. When problems come up, have faith that something good will come out of them. Ask G-d to help you see the good. Look for the good in yourself. Don't dwell on your shortcomings or on what you don't have. Think about your positive points and what you do have!

Honesty and truth: Be realistic: don't pretend that the things you don't want to confront are not there. Facing problems honestly is better than letting them fester and grow more complicated. Don't deceive yourself about who and what you really are - you will only spend a lot of effort maintaining your illusions. Being truthful with yourself does not mean you have to be harshly self-critical: know your good points and be thankful for them.

A Little: Small, tangible gains are better than swollen ambitions and heavy failures. Instead of trying to achieve too much too quickly, do one thing at a time and be content with steady progress in the right direction. What you do today takes you further ahead than what you dream about doing tomorrow. Live in the present moment and make each day into a project on its own - make a success of today!

Patience: Usually, the more valuable the goal, the greater the obstacles which stand in the way of achieving it. Don't be discouraged if things go against you or your efforts seem to be frustrated. If what you want is G-d's will, failure is only a preparation for success: nothing will stop you from achieving what you want in the end. If it is not G-d's will, it would in any case be no good for you in the long run.

Starting: Be willing to learn and change. Nothing obliges you to act out old patterns of behavior just because you followed them until now. The past is gone. Forget about previous failures and make a whole new start. Don't worry if you fall down again. Just pick yourself up and start again, even if you have to do so many times. Every little effort you make is taking you closer to your goal.

"If you will surely *hear* the voice of HaShem your G-d. and listen to His commandments, *all the diseases that I have put upon the Egyptians, I will not put upon you, for I, HaShem am your Healer*" (Exodus 15:26).